"The Vagus Nerve Code: Harnessing the Healing Power Within"

Understanding and Harnessing the Transformative Energy of the Vagus Nerve for Optimal Health and Well-being

By

Dr. Walter M. Price

Table of Contents

CHAPTER ONE

1.0. Introduction to the Vagus Nerve

The human body is composed of countless intricate systems working together to maintain our overall health and well-being. One such system that has gained significant attention in recent years is the vagus nerve. Often referred to as the "wandering nerve," the vagus nerve is the longest cranial nerve in our body, extending from the brainstem all the way down to the abdomen.

The vagus nerve plays a vital role in our overall health by connecting the brain to various organs, including the heart, lungs, stomach, and intestines. It is responsible for regulating important bodily functions such as digestion, heart rate, breathing, and even our mood.

In recent years, researchers and medical professionals have begun to recognize the significant impact that the vagus nerve has on our overall well-being. It has become evident that accessing and stimulating the healing power of the vagus nerve can have profound effects on our physical health, emotional well-being, and mental state.

This book aims to provide a comprehensive understanding of the vagus nerve's functions and its connection to our mind and body. Throughout the following chapters, we will explore various techniques and practices that can be used to activate and harness the healing power of the vagus nerve.

By understanding how the vagus nerve operates and utilizing techniques to stimulate its activity, we can potentially enhance our overall health and well-being. From deep breathing exercises to specific lifestyle changes, we will delve into various approaches that can promote vagus nerve activation and optimize its healing potential.

Furthermore, we will explore the role of nutrition in vagus nerve health, as well as its connection to mental health conditions such as anxiety, depression, and PTSD. By understanding the intricate relationship between the vagus nerve and our mental well-being, we can explore potential therapies and interventions to support mental health.

Whether you are seeking relief from digestive issues, want to improve your emotional well-being, or are interested in optimizing your overall health, accessing the healing power of the vagus nerve can be a useful asset in your excursion toward well-being.

Join us as we delve into the fascinating world of the vagus nerve and discover how to tap into its healing potential for improved physical, emotional, and mental health.

1.1. Overview of Vagus Nerve

The vagus nerve, also known as the tenth cranial nerve, is the longest and most important nerve in the autonomic nervous system. It runs from the brainstem to various organs in the body, including the heart, lungs, stomach, and intestines. The vagus nerve plays a crucial role in regulating many bodily functions, including digestion, heart rate, breathing, and immune responses.

The vagus nerve contains both sensory and motor fibers, allowing it to transmit signals between the brain and various organs. It carries information from the body's organs back to the brain, providing feedback on their status and function. Additionally, it sends signals from the brain to the organs, controlling their activities.

Activation of the vagus nerve has been found to have numerous beneficial effects on health and well-being. It helps to reduce inflammation in the body, lower heart rate and blood pressure, improve digestion and promote relaxation and calmness. The vagus nerve is also involved in the regulation of the body's stress response, and its stimulation can help reduce anxiety and promote a sense of well-being.

There are various techniques and practices that can stimulate the vagus nerve, such as deep breathing exercises, meditation, yoga, and certain types of physical activity. These practices can help harness the healing power within the vagus nerve and promote overall health and well-being. Ongoing research is uncovering the potential of vagus nerve stimulation as a therapeutic approach for conditions such as epilepsy, depression, and chronic pain.

In summary, the vagus nerve plays a vital role in maintaining our body's balance and regulating many important physiological functions. Understanding and harnessing the power of the vagus nerve can have significant implications for our physical health, mental well-being, and overall quality of life.

1.2. Functions of Vagus Nerve

The vagus nerve is involved in a wide range of functions, influencing both the body and the brain. The main functions are as follows:

1. Parasympathetic Control: The vagus nerve is a major component of the parasympathetic nervous system, which is responsible for promoting relaxation, digestion, and restorative processes in the body. It helps to regulate heart rate, respiratory rate, and gastrointestinal functions.

2. Heart Rate and Blood Pressure Regulation: The vagus nerve plays a crucial role in regulating heart rate, specifically by slowing it down. It helps to maintain heart rate variability, which is important for cardiovascular health. The vagus nerve also helps to regulate blood pressure by influencing the dilation and constriction of blood vessels.

3. Gastrointestinal Control: The vagus nerve is a key player in the regulation of digestion and gastrointestinal functions. It stimulates the production of digestive enzymes, enhances gastrointestinal motility, and regulates the release of stomach acids. The vagus nerve also acts as a communication pathway between the gut and the brain, influencing appetite, satiety, and food preference.

4. Respiratory Function: The vagus nerve controls the muscles responsible for respiratory processes, including the diaphragm and other muscles involved in breathing. It helps to regulate the depth and rate of breathing and is involved in maintaining respiratory stability.

5. Immune System Regulation: The vagus nerve has been found to have an anti-inflammatory effect on the body. It can regulate the immune response by inhibiting the release of pro-inflammatory molecules and promoting the release of anti-inflammatory molecules. This makes the vagus nerve a key regulator of the body's immune system.

6. Stress Response and Emotional Regulation: The vagus nerve is involved in the regulation of the body's stress response. It plays a role in calming and resetting the body after a stressor. The vagus nerve also has connections with brain regions associated with emotions and is involved in mood regulation. Stimulation of the vagus nerve has been found to reduce anxiety and promote feelings of relaxation and well-being.

Note: *These are just a few of the many functions of the vagus nerve. It is a complex and important nerve that has widespread effects throughout the body, influencing various physiological processes and contributing to overall health and well-being.*

1.3 Importance of Accessing the Healing Power of the Vagus Nerve

Assessing the healing power of the vagus nerve is crucial for several reasons:

- **Understanding the Body's Innate Healing Mechanisms:** The vagus nerve plays a vital role in the body's self-regulation and healing processes. By assessing its healing power, we gain insights into the body's innate capacity for self-healing and can harness this potential to promote overall health and well-being.

- **Holistic Approach to Healing:** The vagus nerve connects various systems within the body, such as the nervous system, cardiovascular system, digestive system, and immune system. By assessing the healing power of the vagus nerve, we can adopt a holistic approach to healing that addresses the interconnectedness of these systems and promotes overall balance and well-being.

- **Potential Treatment Approach:** Understanding the healing power of the vagus nerve allows us to explore its potential as a treatment approach for various health conditions. Vagus nerve stimulation has shown promising results in the management of conditions such as epilepsy, depression, inflammation, chronic pain, and gastrointestinal disorders. By assessing and harnessing the healing power of the vagus nerve, we can develop targeted interventions that support these therapeutic applications.

- **Enhancing Personal Well-being:** The vagus nerve is involved in mood regulation, stress management, and emotional resilience. By assessing the healing power of the vagus nerve, individuals can gain a better understanding of their own physiological and emotional well-being. This self-awareness allows for the adoption of specific techniques and practices that stimulate and optimize vagus nerve function, leading to improved overall health and quality of life.

- **Advancing Scientific Knowledge:** Assessing the healing power of the vagus nerve contributes to the broader understanding of human physiology and the intricate workings of the nervous system. It enables researchers and healthcare professionals to uncover new insights and develop innovative interventions that leverage the healing potential of the vagus nerve.

In conclusion, assessing the healing power of the vagus nerve is essential for harnessing its full potential in promoting health, well-being, and the body's natural healing processes. By understanding and optimizing vagus nerve function, we can unlock new avenues for therapeutic interventions and empower individuals to take an active role in their own healing journey.

CHAPTER TWO

2.0. Understanding the mind-body connection

The mind-body connection refers to the dynamic relationship between our thoughts, emotions, beliefs, and attitudes (mind) and our physical health and well-being (body). It recognizes that our mental, emotional, and spiritual state can impact our physical health, and vice versa.

Here are some key aspects of understanding the mind-body connection:

- **Psychoneuroimmunology:** Psychoneuroimmunology is a field of study that explores how our mental and emotional states can influence our immune system and overall health. It investigates the complex interactions between psychological factors, the nervous system, and the immune system, highlighting the bidirectional communication between the mind and the body.

- **Stress and the Mind-Body Connection:** Stress is a significant factor in the mind-body connection. When we experience stress, whether it is physical, emotional, or psychological, our body releases stress hormones like cortisol, which can impact our immune system, digestion, cardiovascular health, and more. Persistent stress can add to the turn of events or intensification of different physical and emotional wellness conditions.

- **Placebo and Nocebo Effects:** The mind-body connection is exemplified by the placebo and nocebo effects. The placebo effect refers to the phenomenon where a person experiences a positive response or improvement in symptoms after receiving a treatment or intervention that has no active therapeutic component. On the other hand, the nocebo effect occurs when negative beliefs or expectations about treatment or intervention lead to the worsening of symptoms or adverse effects. These effects demonstrate the power of our thoughts and beliefs in influencing our physical experiences.

- **Mind-Body Practices:** Various mind-body practices, such as meditation, yoga, deep breathing exercises, and mindfulness, aim to cultivate awareness and promote the mind-body connection. These practices have been shown to reduce stress, improve immune function, enhance emotional well-being, and contribute to overall health and healing.

- **Emotions and Physical Health:** Emotions are an integral part of the mind-body connection. Research has demonstrated the way that our profound state can impact our actual well-being . For example, chronic negative emotions like anger, resentment, or depression have been associated with increased cardiovascular risk, weakened immune function, and other health complications. Conversely, positive emotions like joy, gratitude, and love have been linked to improved overall health and longevity.

Note: Understanding the mind-body connection highlights the importance of taking a holistic approach to health and well-being. It emphasizes the need to address not only physical symptoms and diseases but also the underlying mental, emotional, and spiritual aspects that can influence our health. By nurturing a healthy mind-body connection, we can enhance our overall well-being and promote optimal health.

2.1. The Brain-Gut Connection

The brain-gut connection refers to the bidirectional communication between the brain (central nervous system) and the gut (enteric nervous system), which is often referred to as the "second brain." This connection involves various biochemical, neural, and immune pathways that influence the functioning of both the brain and the gut.

Here are some important aspects of the brain-gut connection:

- **The Vagus Nerve:** A significant component of the brain-gut connection is the vagus nerve, which runs from the brainstem to the abdomen. The vagus nerve facilitates bidirectional communication between the brain and the gut, allowing them to exchange signals and information. The vagus nerve plays a critical role in regulating digestive processes, modulating inflammation, and influencing mood and emotions.

- **Gut Microbiome:** The gut is home to trillions of microorganisms known as the gut microbiome. Emerging research has revealed the crucial role of the gut microbiome in the brain-gut connection. The gut microbiome produces various chemicals and metabolites that can influence brain function, behavior, and mood. Additionally, imbalances in the gut microbiome have been linked to conditions such as irritable bowel syndrome (IBS), depression, and anxiety.

- **The Enteric Nervous System (ENS):** The enteric nervous system refers to the network of neurons embedded in the walls of the gastrointestinal tract. This "second brain" of the gut can operate autonomously, controlling digestion and gut motility. The ENS sends signals to the brain and is influenced by the brain, highlighting the bidirectional communication between the two.

- **Stress and Emotions:** Stress, emotions, and psychological factors can significantly impact the gastrointestinal system. The brain-gut connection allows stress and emotions to influence gut function, causing symptoms such as stomachaches, diarrhea, or constipation. On the other hand, gastrointestinal issues can also affect one's emotional well-being. This interconnectedness emphasizes the intimate relationship between mental and digestive health.

- **Impact on Health:** Research has revealed that disturbances in the brain-gut connection can contribute to various gastrointestinal disorders, such as irritable bowel syndrome (IBS), inflammatory bowel disease (IBD), and functional dyspepsia. Additionally, imbalances in the brain-gut connection have been associated with mental health conditions, including anxiety, depression, and even neurodegenerative diseases like Parkinson's disease.

***Note:** Understanding and nurturing the brain-gut connection is essential for maintaining optimal digestive health, promoting emotional well-being, and potentially managing or preventing certain gastrointestinal and mental health conditions. Lifestyle factors such as a healthy diet, regular exercise, stress management techniques, and probiotic supplementation can contribute to a balanced brain-gut connection and overall well-being.*

2.2 The Vagus Nerve and Emotional Well-being

The vagus nerve has a significant impact on emotional well-being and plays a crucial role in regulating mood, emotions, and stress responses.

Here are some key aspects of the relationship between the vagus nerve and emotional well-being:

- **Regulation of the Stress Response:** The vagus nerve is a critical component of the body's parasympathetic nervous system, which helps to counteract the "fight-or-flight" stress response. Activation of the vagus nerve promotes the relaxation response, reduces anxiety, and helps to regulate emotional arousal. It helps to regulate heart rate, blood pressure, and respiration, promoting a sense of calmness and emotional stability.

- **Influence on Emotions:** The vagus nerve has connections with various brain regions involved in emotional processing, including the amygdala, prefrontal cortex, and hippocampus. As a result, the vagus nerve can modulate the intensity and duration of emotional responses. Optimal vagal tone, or the activity of the vagus nerve, is associated with better emotional regulation, greater emotional resilience, and improved overall emotional well-being.

- **Gut-Brain Axis:** The vagus nerve plays a vital role in the bidirectional communication between the gut and the brain. The gut microbiome and the vagus nerve form part of the gut-brain axis, and disruptions in this axis have been associated with mood disorders such as depression and anxiety. The vagus nerve helps to regulate gut function and maintain a healthy gut microbiome, which can influence mood and emotional well-being.

- **Vagus Nerve Stimulation:** Stimulation of the vagus nerve through various techniques, such as deep breathing exercises, mindfulness, and certain medical devices, has been shown to have a positive impact on emotional well-being. Vagus nerve stimulation can reduce anxiety, improve mood, and alleviate symptoms of depression. It is even used as a therapeutic approach for treatment-resistant depression.

- **Heart Rate Variability:** The vagus nerve is involved in regulating heart rate variability (HRV), which is a measure of the variation in the time intervals between heartbeats. Higher HRV is associated with better emotional regulation, resilience to stress, and overall emotional well-being. The vagus nerve helps to maintain healthy HRV, thus contributing to emotional well-being.

Understanding and supporting the vagus nerve's role in emotional well-being can be beneficial for mental health and overall quality of life. By engaging in practices that activate and stimulate the vagus nerve, individuals can enhance their emotional resilience, manage stress more effectively, and promote a greater sense of calmness and well-being.

2.3 How Stress Impacts the Vagus Nerve

Stress can have a significant impact on the function and activity of the vagus nerve. Here's an overview of how stress affects the vagus nerve:

- **Reduced Vagal Tone:** Stress can lead to reduced vagal tone, which refers to the activity and responsiveness of the vagus nerve. Vagal tone is an indicator of the efficiency and effectiveness of the parasympathetic nervous system, which is responsible for promoting relaxation and recovery. During periods of chronic stress, the vagal tone can become suppressed, leading to imbalances in the autonomic nervous system and decreased ability to regulate stress responses.

- **Activation of the Sympathetic Nervous System:** When we experience stress, the body's sympathetic nervous system, which is responsible for the "fight-or-flight" response, becomes activated. This activation can override the activity of the vagus nerve and shift the body into a state of heightened alertness, increased heart rate, rapid breathing, and reduced digestive processes.

- **Impact on Heart Rate Variability (HRV):** Stress can disrupt heart rate variability (HRV), which is a measure of the variation in the time intervals between heartbeats. Higher HRV is associated with better stress resilience and overall health. Chronic stress can lead to reduced HRV, reflecting diminished vagal influence on heart rate modulation.

- **Gut-Brain Axis Dysregulation:** Stress can also disrupt the communication between the gut and the brain, which is regulated by the vagus nerve. Chronic stress can lead to alterations in the gut microbiome, increased gut permeability, and changes in gut motility, all of which can impact emotional well-being and contribute to conditions such as irritable bowel syndrome (IBS) or other gastrointestinal issues.

- **Emotional Regulation:** The vagus nerve plays a role in emotional regulation and dampening the stress response. Chronic stress can impair this process, making it more challenging to regulate emotions effectively and increasing susceptibility to anxiety, depression, and other mental health issues.

It's important to note that while stress can negatively impact the vagus nerve, interventions aimed at reducing stress and promoting relaxation can have a positive effect on vagal tone and overall well-being. Engaging in stress-reducing practices like deep breathing exercises, mindfulness, yoga, and relaxation techniques can help support and restore the activity of the vagus nerve, improving its ability to modulate stress responses and promote emotional well-being.

CHAPTER THREE

3.0. Techniques to Activate the Vagus Nerve

Activating the vagus nerve can have a positive impact on overall well-being and help reduce stress and anxiety.

Here are some techniques to activate the vagus nerve:

1. Deep Breathing: Deep breathing is a technique that helps activate the vagus nerve, which is fundamental in promoting relaxation and reducing stress. Engaging in deep, diaphragmatic breathing helps stimulate the vagus nerve. Breathe in slowly through your nose, allowing your diaphragm to expand fully, and exhale slowly through your mouth.

Here's a detailed explanation of the process:

- **Find a comfortable position:** Begin by finding a comfortable seated position, either on a chair or on the floor with your back straight and shoulders relaxed.

- **Relax your body:** Close your eyes and take a moment to mentally scan your body for any tension. consciously release any tension you may feel in your muscles, especially in your neck, shoulders, and jaw.

- **Inhale slowly through your nose:** Take a slow, deep breath in through your nose, imagining your diaphragm expanding and your belly rising. Allow the breath to fill your lungs completely as much as possible.

- **Pause briefly:** Once you have inhaled fully, briefly pause for a moment, holding your breath in gently.

- **Exhale slowly through your mouth:** Begin to exhale slowly through your mouth, imagining your breath flowing out smoothly and evenly. Allow the exhale to be longer than the inhale, aiming for a slow and controlled release of breath.

- **Repeat the process:** Continue this deep breathing technique, taking slow and deep breaths in through your nose, briefly pausing, and then exhaling slowly through your mouth. Aim to make each breath steady and rhythmic.

- **Focus on your breath:** As you continue deep breathing, bring your attention to the sensation of the breath entering and leaving your body. Notice the rise and fall of your belly or the coolness of the air entering your nostrils. Try to stay present and focused on breathing throughout the exercise.

- **Practice for a few minutes:** Start with a few minutes of deep breathing and gradually increase the duration as you become more comfortable with the technique. You can set a timer or simply practice until you feel a sense of calm and relaxation.

By engaging in deep breathing, you are activating the vagus nerve, which is responsible for activating the parasympathetic nervous system—the "rest-and-digest" response. This helps counteract the effects of stress and promotes a sense of relaxation and well-being. Deep breathing not only helps activate the vagus nerve but also increases oxygen levels in the body, lowers heart rate, and reduces blood pressure, further enhancing the relaxation response.

2. Cold Exposure: Cold exposure is a technique that can activate the vagus nerve by stimulating the body's fight-or-flight response. Exposing yourself to cold temperatures, such as taking cold showers or ice baths, has been shown to activate the vagus nerve. The shock of the cold stimulates the body's fight-or-flight response, which in turn activates the vagus nerve.

Here's a detailed explanation of the process:

- **Cold showers or baths:** Cold exposure can be achieved by taking cold showers or immersing yourself in cold water. Start by adjusting the water temperature gradually, beginning with warm water and gradually decreasing the temperature. You can also try plunging into a cold pool or taking an ice bath.

- **Initial shock:** As your body first comes into contact with the cold water, you will likely experience a shock or gasping sensation. This is a natural response to the sudden change in temperature and stimulates the body's fight-or-flight response, which activates the sympathetic nervous system.

- **Breathing and relaxation:** Despite the initial shock, try to remain calm and maintain control over your breathing. Take slow, full breaths and spotlight on loosening up your body. This helps activate the vagus nerve and the parasympathetic branch of the autonomic nervous system, promoting a sense of relaxation and well-being.

- **Gradual exposure:** Start with short durations of cold exposure, such as 30 seconds, and gradually increase the time as you become more accustomed to the cold. In any case, it's essential to pay attention to your body and not propel yourself past your cutoff points. If you feel uncomfortable or experience any adverse reactions, discontinue the cold exposure.

- **Repeated exposure:** Consistency is key when it comes to cold exposure. Try to incorporate this practice into your routine regularly, such as taking cold showers or baths daily or a few times a week. Over time, your body will become more tolerant of the cold, and the activation of the vagus nerve will become more efficient.

- **Cold exposure alternatives:** If immersing yourself in cold water is not feasible or comfortable for you, there are other methods of cold exposure. This includes using cold packs or ice packs on specific areas of your body, immersing your face in cold water, or even stepping outside in cold weather for a short period.

NOTE: *Cold exposure activates the vagus nerve through the stimulation of the body's stress response and subsequent activation of the sympathetic nervous system. However, it's important to note that cold exposure may not be suitable for everyone, especially those with underlying health conditions or compromised immune systems. It's always best to consult with a* *medical care proficient prior to integrating any new practices into your daily schedule.*

3. Singing or Chanting: Vocal exercises like singing or chanting can activate the vagus nerve. These activities involve controlled breathing and vocalization, both of which stimulate the functions of the nerve.

The vagus nerve is the longest cranial nerve in the human body, and it plays a crucial role in regulating many bodily functions such as heart rate, digestion, and respiration. It is also known to be involved in calming the body and reducing stress.

The singing or chanting of the vagus nerve involves using specific vocal techniques to stimulate and activate this nerve. It is based on the understanding that the vagus nerve is closely connected to the muscles of the throat and vocal cords. By manipulating the vocal cords through singing or chanting, one can indirectly stimulate the vagus nerve.

Here is a detailed explanation of how singing or chanting activates the vagus nerve:

- **Deep breathing:** Singing or chanting typically involves deep breathing techniques, which help to increase the oxygen flow to the brain and stimulate the vagus nerve. Deep breathing also helps to slow down the heart rate, lower blood pressure, and activate the parasympathetic nervous system, which is controlled by the vagus nerve.

- **Vocalization:** Singing or chanting requires controlled and deliberate vocalization. The vibrations produced by vocal cords during singing stimulate the vagus nerve. These vibrations travel through the middle ear and reach the cranial nerves, including the vagus nerve, thereby activating it.

- **Long tones or sustained vocalization:** Singing or chanting often involves holding long tones or sustained vocalizations. This prolonged vocalization activates the muscles of the throat and vocal cords for an extended period, providing consistent stimulation to the vagus nerve.

- **Resonation:** Certain vocal techniques emphasize resonation, which refers to the amplification and vibration of sound in the cranial and facial bones. Resonation helps to further stimulate the vagus nerve by enhancing the vibrations that reach the nerves in the head and throat.

- **Neural synchronization:** Singing or chanting in groups or with others can enhance the effects on the vagus nerve. When multiple individuals engage in synchronized singing or chanting, the neural activity in their brains becomes more coordinated and harmonized. This synchronization has been shown to increase vagal tone, which is an indicator of the activity and effectiveness of the vagus nerve.

- **Emotional regulation:** Singing or chanting has been known to induce positive emotions and relaxation. When we engage in these activities, the brain releases endorphins and oxytocin, which promote feelings of happiness, pleasure, and bonding. These positive emotions further activate the vagus nerve and contribute to its calming and stress-reducing effects.

- **Mind-body connection:** Singing or chanting often involves a focus on mindfulness and the mind-body connection. By directing our attention to the sensations and vibrations in our bodies while singing or chanting, we can enhance the activation of the vagus nerve. This mindful awareness helps to deepen the connection between the brain and the body, facilitating the regulation of bodily functions by the vagus nerve.

In summary, singing or chanting of the vagus nerve involves using specific vocal techniques to stimulate and activate the nerve. Deep breathing, vocalization, sustained vocal tones, resonation, neural synchronization, emotional regulation, and mind-body connection are key elements of this practice. By engaging in these activities, we can enhance the function of the vagus nerve, leading to relaxation, stress reduction, and improved overall well-being.

4. Meditation: Practicing mindfulness meditation or other forms of relaxation exercises can activate the vagus nerve. The focused attention and deep relaxation achieved during meditation activate the parasympathetic branch of the nervous system, where the vagus nerve plays a crucial role.

The meditation of the vagus nerve involves specific techniques that are designed to activate and stimulate this important cranial nerve. The vagus nerve plays a crucial role in regulating various bodily functions, including heart rate, digestion, respiration, and stress response. By focusing on the vagus nerve during meditation, we can activate its calming effects and promote overall well-being.

Here is a detailed explanation of how to meditate on the vagus nerve:

- **Find a comfortable position:** Start by finding a comfortable seated or lying position. Shut your eyes and loosen up your body.

- **Deep breathing:** Begin by taking slow, deep breaths. Breathe in profoundly through your nose, permitting your tummy to grow, and breathe out leisurely through your mouth. Deep breathing activates the parasympathetic nervous system, which is controlled by the vagus nerve, and helps to promote relaxation and stress reduction.

- **Focus on the breath:** Direct your attention to the sensations of your breath. Notice the ebb and flow of your breath as you inhale and exhale.

Stay present with each breath, observing the gentle rise and fall of your abdomen or the coolness and warmth of the breath at your nostrils.

- **Lengthen the exhale:** As you continue to breathe deeply and focus on your breath, consciously lengthen your exhale. Extend the duration of your exhale, making it slightly longer than your inhale. This extended exhale helps to activate the vagus nerve and stimulate its calming effects on the body.

- **Use affirmations or mantras:** While focusing on your breath, you can incorporate affirmations or mantras that are specifically designed to activate the vagus nerve. Phrases such as "I am calm and relaxed" or "I am safe and at peace" can be repeated silently or out loud during your meditation practice. These affirmations help to reinforce a sense of safety, tranquility, and well-being, further stimulating the vagus nerve.

- **Visualize the vagus nerve:** During your meditation practice, you can visualize the vagus nerve running through your body. Imagine it as a long, delicate, and vibrant nerve that extends from your brainstem down to your abdomen. Visualizing the vagus nerve helps to strengthen the connection between your mind and body, enhancing the effects of meditation on the nerve.

- **Body awareness:** Expand your awareness beyond your breath and focus on the sensations in different parts of your body. Check your body from head to toe, seeing any areas of pressure or distress. As you come across areas of tension, bring your attention to those areas and consciously relax them. This body awareness helps to promote the activation of the vagus nerve by bringing attention and relaxation to different parts of the body that may be holding stress or tension.

- **Practice gratitude and loving-kindness:** Incorporate gratitude and loving-kindness into your meditation practice. As you continue to breathe deeply and focus on the vagus nerve, bring to mind moments of gratitude and think of people or things you are grateful for. Additionally, cultivate feelings of compassion and send wishes for well-being and happiness to yourself and others. These positive emotions further activate the vagus nerve and contribute to its calming and soothing effects.

Extend the meditation practice: Aim to maintain your meditation practice for at least 10-15 minutes, but feel free to extend it for longer periods if you have time. Consistency in practice is key for the benefits of vagus nerve meditation to be experienced fully.

By incorporating these techniques into your meditation practice, you can activate and stimulate the vagus nerve, promoting relaxation, stress reduction, and overall well-being. Regular practice will help strengthen the mind-body connection and enhance the benefits of meditating on the vagus nerve.

NOTE: *While this information is based on scientific understanding and anecdotal evidence, it is always important to consult with a healthcare professional or qualified meditation instructor before starting any* *new meditation or relaxation practices. They can provide personalized guidance and ensure that it is safe and appropriate for your individual needs.*

5. Yoga: Certain yoga poses, such as the cobra pose and the fish pose, are known to stimulate the vagus nerve. These poses stretch and compress specific areas of the body, activating the nerve and increasing its tone.

The yoga of the vagus nerve involves a series of yoga poses, breathing techniques, and mindfulness practices that are specifically designed to activate and stimulate the vagus nerve. The vagus nerve is the longest cranial nerve in the body and plays a key role in regulating various bodily functions, including heart rate, digestion, respiratory function, and stress response. By engaging in yoga practices that target the vagus nerve, we can promote relaxation, reduce stress, and enhance overall well-being.

Here is a detailed explanation of how to practice yoga for the vagus nerve:

- **Deep breathing exercises:** Begin your yoga practice by focusing on deep breathing. Practice diaphragmatic breathing, also known as belly breathing, which involves breathing deeply into your belly, expanding it on the inhale, and contracting it on the exhale. Deep breathing activates the parasympathetic nervous system, which is controlled by the vagus nerve, and helps to induce a state of relaxation.

- **Chest-opening poses:** Engage in yoga poses that open and expand the chest, such as the Cobra pose (Bhujangasana), Bridge pose (Setu Bandha Sarvangasana), or Fish pose (Matsyasana). These poses stretch the muscles around the chest, ribcage, and throat, providing a gentle stimulation to the vagus nerve. They also help to improve respiratory function and enhance the flow of oxygen to the brain.

- **Neck stretches:** Incorporate gentle stretches and movements for the neck. Neck rolls, side-to-side neck stretches, and gentle neck tilts help to release tension and improve circulation in the neck area where the vagus nerve runs. These movements can help to stimulate the vagus nerve indirectly.

- **Restorative poses:** Include restorative yoga poses in your practice that encourage deep relaxation and rest. Poses such as Legs-Up-The-Wall (Viparita Karani),

Child's Pose (Balasana), or Corpse Pose (Savasana) allow for a comfortable and supported position that promotes a sense of calmness and activates the parasympathetic nervous system.

- **Chanting and humming:** Incorporate vocalization practices into your yoga practice, such as chanting or humming. Chanting specific sounds such as "Om" or "Aum" and humming vibrations create resonance in the throat and activate the vagus nerve. These practices enhance the mind-body connection and promote relaxation.

- **Mindfulness meditation:** Integrate mindfulness meditation into your yoga practice. Mindfulness involves bringing awareness to the present moment and observing sensations, thoughts, and emotions without judgment. By cultivating mindfulness during yoga, we can enhance our connection with the body and further stimulate the vagus nerve. Focus on the breath, bring attention to the physical sensations of each pose, and observe how the body responds during the practice.

- **Balancing poses:** Engage in balancing yoga poses, such as Tree pose (Vrksasana) or Eagle pose (Garudasana), which require focus and concentration. Balancing poses help to activate the vagus nerve by engaging the parasympathetic nervous system and promoting a sense of balance and stability.

- **Savasana and guided relaxation:** Finish your yoga practice with Savasana (Corpse Pose) or guided relaxation techniques. Lie down on your back, allowing your body to fully relax and integrate the benefits of your yoga practice. Guided relaxation techniques, such as body scans or progressive muscle relaxation, promote deep relaxation and further activate the vagus nerve.

Consistency in practicing yoga for the vagus nerve is key to experiencing the benefits fully. Aim for regular practice, at least a few times a week, and gradually increase the duration and intensity of your practice over time. Listen to your body and practice within your own abilities and comfort level.

NOTE: *It is important to note that practicing yoga for the vagus nerve should be done mindfully and with awareness of your body's needs and* *limitations. If you have any pre-existing health conditions or concerns, it is always recommended to consult with a healthcare professional or a qualified yoga instructor before starting a new yoga practice.*

By incorporating these yoga practices into your routine, you can activate and stimulate the vagus nerve, promoting relaxation, stress reduction, and overall well-being. Yoga offers a holistic approach to connecting the mind, body, and spirit, and it can have profound effects on the functioning of the vagus nerve and the regulation of bodily functions.

6. Vagus Nerve Stimulation Devices: There are specialized devices available, such as vagus nerve stimulators, that can directly stimulate the vagus nerve. These devices are typically used in medical settings for specific conditions, but they can also be utilized as a form of therapy under professional guidance.

Vagus Nerve Stimulation (VNS) devices are medical devices designed to deliver electrical stimulation to the vagus nerve, which runs from the brainstem to various organs in the body. VNS devices are approved by regulatory authorities for the treatment of specific medical conditions such as epilepsy, depression, and migraines.

Here is a detailed explanation of Vagus Nerve Stimulation devices:

- **Implantable VNS Devices:** These are the most common type of VNS devices and require a surgical procedure to implant the device under the skin in the chest area. The device consists of a generator, electrodes, and a lead wire that is connected to the vagus nerve. The generator is programmable and delivers regular electrical impulses to the vagus nerve, typically on a predetermined schedule. The intensity and frequency of the impulses can be adjusted by a healthcare professional based on individual needs. The electrical stimulation activates the vagus nerve, which in turn affects the functions regulated by the nerve, such as reducing the frequency of seizures in epilepsy patients.

- **External VNS Devices:** Unlike implantable VNS devices, external VNS devices do not require surgery and are worn externally on the body. These devices typically consist of a handheld or wearable stimulator that delivers electrical impulses to the vagus nerve through electrodes placed on the skin. The electrodes are usually positioned over the neck area, where the vagus nerve is located. Similar to the implantable devices, the external VNS devices deliver electrical stimulation to the vagus nerve, providing therapeutic benefits for conditions such as depression or migraines. External VNS devices are usually used in a clinical or hospital setting under the guidance of healthcare professionals.

- **Non-invasive VNS Devices:** Non-invasive VNS devices are the latest innovation in VNS therapy. They do not require any surgery or placement of electrodes on the skin. Instead, these devices use alternative methods to stimulate the vagus nerve. For example, some non-invasive VNS devices use transcutaneous electrical nerve stimulation (TENS) technology, where electrical impulses are delivered through the skin to stimulate the vagus nerve without the need for invasive procedures. Other non-invasive VNS devices may use magnetic fields to stimulate the nerve. These devices are still relatively new and are being studied for their efficacy in various conditions.

It is important to note that VNS devices should be used under the guidance and supervision of healthcare professionals who can determine the appropriate settings, frequencies, and intensity levels based on the individual's condition and needs. Only healthcare providers can prescribe and properly assess the suitability of VNS devices for specific medical conditions.

VNS devices, whether implantable, external, or non-invasive, are designed to provide therapeutic benefits by modulating the activity of the vagus nerve. The precise mechanism of action is still being studied, but it is believed that the electrical stimulation of the vagus nerve can affect neurotransmitter release, brain activity, and various physiological functions.

While VNS devices have shown promising results in treating certain medical conditions, they may also carry potential risks and side effects. Common side effects include hoarseness, cough, shortness of breath, and discomfort around the implanted site. Some individuals may experience more serious side effects such as infection or vocal cord paralysis. Additionally, certain precautions and contraindications may apply, and individuals with medical devices such as pacemakers or defibrillators may require special considerations.

It is always important to consult with a healthcare professional or specialist to discuss the benefits, risks, and suitability of VNS devices for specific medical conditions. They can provide personalized guidance, monitor device settings, and ensure proper follow-up care to maximize the therapeutic benefits and minimize potential risks associated with VNS therapy.

__NOTE:__ Please note that the information provided here is for educational purposes only and should not be considered as medical advice. If you have any questions or concerns about Vagus Nerve Stimulation devices or their suitability for your specific condition, please consult with a healthcare professional.

7. Laughter: Genuine laughter has been found to activate the vagus nerve. Engaging in activities that induce laughter, such as watching a funny movie or telling jokes, can help stimulate the nerve and promote overall well-being.

The "laughter of the vagus nerve" refers to the physiological and psychological benefits of laughter on the function of the vagus nerve. The vagus nerve, otherwise called the "meandering nerve," is the longest cranial nerve in the body. It is responsible for regulating many bodily functions, including heart rate, digestion, and respiration. It also plays a role in the body's stress response and the activation of the parasympathetic nervous system.

When we laugh genuinely and deeply, it has a positive impact on the vagus nerve in several ways:

- **Increased heart rate variability:** Laughter stimulates the parasympathetic nervous system, which is controlled by the vagus nerve. The parasympathetic sensory system advances unwinding and dials back the pulse. Laughter triggers irregular and rhythmic variations in heart rate, known as heart rate variability (HRV). Increased HRV is associated with better cardiovascular health and overall well-being.

- **Improved mood and stress reduction:** Laughter triggers the release of beneficial hormones, such as endorphins and dopamine, which are associated with pleasure, happiness, and stress reduction. These hormonal changes activate the vagus nerve, leading to a sense of relaxation and improved mood.

- **Enhanced digestion**: The vagus nerve is closely connected to many organs involved in digestion, including the stomach, intestines, liver, and pancreas. When we laugh, the rhythmic contractions of the diaphragm and abdominal muscles stimulate the vagus nerve, promoting better digestion and nutrient absorption. Laughter can also help to alleviate gastrointestinal symptoms related to stress, such as indigestion or stomachaches.

- **Improved lung function:** During laughter, deep inhalation and exhalation occur, involving the activation of the respiratory muscles and the expansion of the lungs. This deep breathing pattern stimulates the vagus nerve and increases oxygen intake, leading to better lung function and improved respiratory health.

- **Enhanced immune function:** The vagus nerve plays a role in regulating the immune system by communicating between the brain and immune cells. Laughter activates the vagus nerve, which, in turn, stimulates the release of cytokines, chemical messengers that regulate immune function. This can lead to a temporary boost in immune activity, enhancing the body's defense against infections and illness.

- **Pain relief:** Laughter has been found to have analgesic effects, reducing pain sensitivity. This pain relief response is partly attributed to the activation of the vagus nerve, which modulates pain perception.

- **Social bonding and connection:** Laughter is a social behavior that promotes bonding and connection with others. When we laugh together, it releases oxytocin, often referred to as the "love hormone," which enhances feelings of trust and connection. This social bonding aspect of laughter further activates the vagus nerve, promoting a sense of well-being and improved social interactions.

In summary, the laughter of the vagus nerve refers to the positive effects of laughter on the functioning of the vagus nerve. Genuine laughter stimulates the parasympathetic nervous system, improves heart rate variability, reduces stress, enhances mood, aids digestion, improves lung function, boosts immune activity, provides pain relief, and promotes social bonding. These benefits demonstrate the powerful connection between laughter, the activation of the vagus nerve, and overall well-being. So, go ahead and embrace laughter as a natural and enjoyable way to enhance the functioning of your vagus nerve and improve your health and happiness.

8. Acupuncture: Acupuncture, a traditional Chinese medicine practice that involves inserting thin needles into specific points on the body, has been found to stimulate the vagus nerve. By stimulating these acupuncture points, the nerve is activated, leading to various health benefits.

When performing acupuncture of the vagus nerve, an acupuncturist closely follows the pathway of the nerve and identifies specific acupuncture points to stimulate. These points may be located on the neck, behind the ear, or on other parts of the body along the nerve pathway. The choice of points depends on the specific condition being addressed and the desired therapeutic effect.

The stimulation of these acupuncture points activates sensory receptors, which send signals to the brain and trigger various mechanisms. Acupuncture of the vagus nerve is believed to stimulate the parasympathetic nervous system, which is responsible for the "rest-and-digest" response in the body. This assists with balancing the impacts of the thoughtful sensory system, which is answerable for the "survival" reaction.

Acupuncture of the vagus nerve has been studied for its potential therapeutic benefits in several conditions, including chronic pain, depression, anxiety, digestive disorders, and inflammatory conditions. The stimulation of the vagus nerve through acupuncture is thought to release neurotransmitters such as serotonin and dopamine, which are involved in mood regulation and pain modulation. It may also help to balance the autonomic nervous system, reduce inflammation, and improve blood flow to affected areas.

During an acupuncture session targeting the vagus nerve, the acupuncturist will first conduct a thorough evaluation to understand the individual's medical history, symptoms, and desired outcomes. They will then determine the appropriate acupuncture points to be stimulated. The acupuncturist will sterilize the skin and use thin, sterile needles to gently insert them into the identified points. The needles are usually left in place for a specific period, typically around 20-30 minutes. The patient may experience a mild sensation of tingling, warmth, or pressure at the insertion sites, but acupuncture is generally considered to be a painless procedure.

The frequency and duration of acupuncture treatments targeting the vagus nerve can vary depending on the individual and the condition being treated. Some patients may experience immediate relief or improvement after a single session, while others may require multiple sessions over a period of weeks or months for optimal results.

It is important to note that while acupuncture of the vagus nerve can be a valuable adjunctive therapy, it should not replace conventional medical treatments. It is constantly prescribed to talk with a certified medical services proficient prior to beginning any new therapy or treatment.

In summary, acupuncture of the vagus nerve involves stimulating specific acupuncture points along the path of the vagus nerve to regulate its function and promote overall health and wellness. By modulating the activity of the vagus nerve, acupuncture can influence several bodily functions and has been studied for its potential benefits in various conditions. However, more research is needed to fully understand the mechanisms and effectiveness of acupuncture for vagus nerve stimulation.

9. Massage: Massaging certain areas of the body, particularly the neck, can stimulate the vagus nerve. Gentle pressure or circular motions applied to the neck area can help activate the nerve and promote relaxation.

Activating the vagus nerve can help reduce stress, promote relaxation, and improve overall well-being.

There are several massage techniques that can be used to stimulate the vagus nerve, including:

1. Neck Massage:

- Begin by sitting or lying comfortably with relaxed shoulders.

- Use your fingertips to apply gentle pressure along the sides of the neck, starting from the base of the skull and moving downward.
- Slowly and gently massage the sides of the neck using circular or kneading motions.
- Continue to apply moderate pressure while moving your fingertips in a downward motion towards the chest.

This massage technique helps release tension in the neck muscles and can indirectly stimulate the vagus nerve.

2. Deep Breathing:

- Deep breathing is an effective way to stimulate the vagus nerve and activate the parasympathetic nervous system.
- Allow your breath to deepen naturally, taking slow and controlled breaths in

through your nose and out through your mouth.

- As you inhale, focus on expanding your diaphragm and filling your lungs completely.
- Exhale slowly, counting to at least four to ensure you are activating the relaxation response.

Repeat this deep breathing technique for several minutes, focusing on lengthening the exhale and allowing the body to relax.

3. Auricular (Ear) Massage:

- The vagus nerve has connections in the ear, making auricular massage an effective way to activate it.
- Gently massage the outer part of the ear using circular motions with your thumb and index finger.
- Start at the top of the ear and gradually work your way down, paying

attention to any tender or sensitive points.

- You can also apply gentle pressure to the earlobe and move it in a circular motion.

Auricular massage can help stimulate the vagus nerve and promote relaxation.

4. Abdominal Massage:

- The vagus nerve innervates many organs in the abdomen, making abdominal massage a powerful technique to activate it.
- Lie down and relax your body, ensuring that your abdomen is uncovered and accessible.
- Use gentle circular motions with your fingertips or palm to massage your abdomen.

- Begin at the center of your abdomen, just below the rib cage, and gradually move in a clockwise direction.
- Apply gentle pressure and focus on relaxing your abdomen, allowing any tension or stress to melt away.

Abdominal massage can help stimulate digestion, improve blood flow, and activate the parasympathetic response through the vagus nerve.

NOTE: *While these massage techniques can help activate the vagus nerve, they should be performed with care and mindfulness. If you have any underlying medical conditions or concerns, it is recommended to consult with a healthcare practitioner before trying these techniques. Additionally, it is always advised to seek the guidance of a qualified massage therapist for more specific and targeted massage techniques to stimulate the vagus nerve.*

10. Exercise: Engaging in moderate-intensity exercises like walking, jogging, or cycling can activate the vagus nerve. Regular physical activity has been shown to enhance the vagal tone, which is an indicator of the vagus nerve's health and efficiency.

There are several exercises that can help to tone and strengthen the vagus nerve. One such exercise is deep and slow breathing. Taking in deep breaths, holding them, and then exhaling slowly helps activate the vagus nerve and initiates the relaxation response in the body. This exercise can be done by taking a deep breath in through the nose, holding it for a few seconds, and then slowly releasing the breath through the mouth. Repeat this process several times to stimulate the vagus nerve.

Another exercise that activates the vagus nerve is singing or chanting. These activities involve controlled breathing, vocalization, and increased expiratory force, which can all help stimulate the vagus nerve and promote relaxation. Singing or chanting can be done alone or in a group and can be as simple as humming a tune or reciting a mantra.

Gargling with water is another exercise that stimulates the vagus nerve. Gargling involves the muscles in the back of the throat and activates the vagus nerve, leading to a sense of relaxation and well-being. To perform this exercise, fill your mouth with water and tilt your head back slightly. Then, make a "gurgling" sound by forcing air and water to move back and forth in the back of your throat. Repeat this exercise several times for maximum benefit.

Cold exposure is also an effective way to stimulate the vagus nerve. Cold showers or plunges into ice-cold water can activate the body's stress response and trigger the release of certain neurotransmitters that stimulate the vagus nerve. The shock of the cold causes the body to activate its natural defense mechanisms and release various chemicals that improve mood, reduce inflammation, and enhance overall well-being.

Lastly, practicing mindfulness and meditation can also have a positive impact on the vagus nerve. These practices involve focusing on the present moment and promoting a sense of calm and relaxation. Mindfulness and meditation help to reduce stress and anxiety levels, allowing the vagus nerve to function optimally. By adopting a regular mindfulness or meditation practice, individuals can train their minds to activate the relaxation response and promote vagal tone.

In conclusion, exercises that stimulate the vagus nerve can have significant benefits for overall well-being. Deep and slow breathing, singing or chanting, gargling with water, cold exposure, and mindfulness and meditation are all effective exercises to activate and strengthen the vagus nerve. Regular practice of these exercises can help regulate bodily functions, reduce stress and anxiety, and promote relaxation and a sense of well-being.

11. Socializing: Spending time with loved ones and engaging in social interactions can stimulate the vagus nerve. Positive social interactions and emotional connections have been shown to increase vagal tone and promote overall well-being.

Socializing of the vagus nerve refers to the influence that social interactions and relationships can have on the functioning of this nerve. The vagus nerve is a key component of the autonomic nervous system, which controls many of the body's involuntary functions. It plays a crucial role in the body's relaxation response, which helps the body calm down after experiencing stress or danger.

When we engage in positive social interactions, such as spending time with loved ones, hugging, or engaging in intimate conversations, it can have a soothing effect on the body. This is due to the socializing of the vagus nerve. Social interactions stimulate the parasympathetic branch of the autonomic nervous system, which is mediated by the vagus nerve. This branch promotes a state of rest and relaxation, counteracting the effects of the sympathetic branch, which is responsible for the body's fight-or-flight response.

When the vagus nerve is activated through socializing, it releases the neurotransmitter acetylcholine, which has various effects on the body. It helps to lower heart rate and blood pressure, promote digestion, and reduce inflammation. It also stimulates the release of oxytocin, often referred to as the "love hormone," which is associated with feelings of trust, social bonding, and well-being.

Socializing of the vagus nerve has been shown to have several positive effects on overall health and well-being. It can help to reduce stress levels, improve mood, and enhance immune function. Studies have also suggested that social interaction and positive social relationships can lower the risk of developing cardiovascular diseases, improve cognitive function, and enhance longevity.

On the other hand, a lack of social interactions or experiencing social isolation can have detrimental effects on the vagus nerve and overall health. Research has linked social isolation to negative health outcomes such as increased inflammation, higher blood pressure, and a higher risk of mental health disorders.

In summary, socializing of the vagus nerve refers to the way social interactions and relationships can positively influence the functioning of this important nerve. By engaging in positive social interactions, we can stimulate the vagus nerve and activate the body's relaxation response, leading to various health benefits. Conversely, a lack of social interactions can be detrimental to the vagus nerve and overall health. Therefore, nurturing social connections and engaging in meaningful social interactions is important for promoting overall well-being.

12. Mindful Eating: Paying attention to the eating process, savoring each bite, and chewing food thoroughly can stimulate the vagus nerve. This mindful eating technique activates the body's rest-and-digest response, which is regulated by the vagus nerve.

Mindful eating refers to the practice of deliberately paying attention to the sensations and experience of eating. When it comes to the vagus nerve, mindful eating can be a powerful tool to improve digestion, reduce stress, and promote overall well-being.

Here's a detailed explanation of how mindful eating can positively impact the vagus nerve:

- **Activation of the parasympathetic nervous system:** The vagus nerve is a critical component of the parasympathetic nervous system, responsible for the body's "rest and digest" response. Mindful eating activates this system by promoting a relaxed state, which stimulates the release of digestive enzymes and enhances nutrient absorption.

- **Improved digestion:** Mindful eating involves slowing down, being present, and savoring the food. This allows the vagus nerve to send signals to the digestive system, helping to regulate stomach acid production, intestinal secretions, and muscle contractions. This, in turn, promotes more efficient digestion and reduces symptoms of indigestion, bloating, and acid reflux.

- **Enhanced satiety and weight management:** Mindful eating helps deepen our awareness of hunger and fullness sensations, allowing us to better regulate our eating. The vagus nerve plays a role in signaling the brain when we are full, sending messages of satiety and reducing the likelihood of overeating. By practicing mindful eating, we can tune into these signals and prevent mindless, excessive consumption, thus supporting weight management and overall health.

- **Reduced stress and anxiety:** The vagus nerve is involved in the regulation of the body's stress response. By engaging in mindful eating, we create a calm and relaxed state, activating the vagus nerve's ability to dampen the stress response.

This can lead to reduced levels of stress hormones, such as cortisol, and promote a sense of well-being.

- **Increased nutrient absorption:** Mindful eating allows us to fully appreciate the taste, texture, and aroma of our food. The vagus nerve plays a role in the release of digestive enzymes and the stimulation of stomach acid production, enhancing our ability to break down and absorb nutrients from the food we consume. When we eat mindfully, we are more likely to thoroughly chew our food, breaking it down into smaller particles for easier digestion and absorption.

To practice mindful eating and engage the vagus nerve effectively, here are some tips:

- **Create a calm environment:** Choose a peaceful and quiet space for your meals. Limit interruptions like TV, telephones, or other electronic gadgets

- **Slow down:** Take your time to eat, savoring each bite. Bite your food completely and focus on the flavors, surfaces, and smells.

- **Tune into your body:** Before you start eating, take a moment to check in with yourself. Notice any hunger or fullness sensations. Throughout the meal, pause occasionally to assess your level of fullness and adjust your eating accordingly.

- **Engage your senses:** Pay attention to the visual aspects of your food, its smell, and how it feels in your mouth. This helps to heighten your awareness and enjoyment of the eating experience.

- **Practice gratitude:** Take a moment to express gratitude for the food in front of you, acknowledging the effort and resources that went into its production. This can cultivate a sense of appreciation and mindfulness.

- **Breathe deeply:** Focus on taking slow, deep breaths while you eat. This helps activate the parasympathetic nervous system and promotes relaxation.

By incorporating these mindful eating practices into your daily routine, you can foster a more harmonious relationship between your body and the vagus nerve, leading to improved digestion, reduced stress and anxiety, and overall well-being.

13. Probiotics: Consuming probiotic-rich foods or taking probiotic supplements can promote a healthy gut microbiome. A healthy gut microbiome has been linked to increased vagus nerve activity and improved overall health.

Probiotics are live bacteria and yeasts that are beneficial for our health, primarily by improving the balance of gut microbiota. Gut microbiota refers to the diverse community of microorganisms residing in our intestinal tract, including both beneficial and harmful bacteria. The gut microbiota has a bidirectional relationship with the central nervous system via the gut-brain axis, and the vagus nerve is a key component of this communication network.

Scientists have been exploring the potential of probiotics to modulate the vagus nerve activity and improve various aspects of health.

Here are a few ways through which probiotics can influence the vagus nerve:

- **Serotonin Production:** Probiotics can produce neurotransmitters such as serotonin, which plays a crucial role in regulating mood and gut motility. Serotonin production in the gut is modulated by the vagus nerve, and disturbances in this pathway can lead to gastrointestinal disorders. Probiotics that promote serotonin production can help regulate gut motility and improve digestive health.

- **Regulation of Inflammation:** Chronic inflammation is associated with many health conditions, including cardiovascular disease and neurodegenerative disorders. The vagus nerve acts as a powerful anti-inflammatory pathway by regulating the release of pro-inflammatory cytokines. Probiotics can modulate the response of the immune system and reduce inflammation by interacting with the vagus nerve.

- **Gut Barrier Function:** The gut barrier refers to the protective lining of the intestinal wall that prevents harmful substances and bacteria from entering the bloodstream. Disruption of the gut barrier can lead to a variety of health issues. Probiotics have been shown to enhance the integrity of the gut barrier by increasing the production of tight junction proteins, which help maintain the tight seal between intestinal cells. The vagus nerve is involved in the regulation of gut barrier function, and probiotics can influence this process by stimulating vagal activity.

- **Neurotransmitter Regulation:** Probiotics can also influence the production and release of neurotransmitters in the gut, such as gamma-aminobutyric acid (GABA) and acetylcholine. GABA is an inhibitory neurotransmitter that helps regulate anxiety and stress levels, while acetylcholine is an excitatory neurotransmitter that plays a role in memory and cognitive function. Both these neurotransmitters are involved in the regulation of the vagus nerve activity. Probiotics that can modulate the production and release of these neurotransmitters can indirectly influence the activity of the vagus nerve.

To harness the benefits of probiotics for the vagus nerve, various techniques can be employed:

- **Choosing the Right Strains:** Different strains of probiotics have different effects on the gut microbiota and the vagus nerve. Lactobacillus and Bifidobacterium species are commonly used probiotics that have been shown to positively influence vagus nerve activity. Therefore, it is important to choose probiotic supplements or foods that contain these specific strains to target vagal modulation.

- **Prebiotics:** Prebiotics are dietary fibers that serve as food for beneficial bacteria in the gut. Consuming prebiotics can promote the growth of specific strains of probiotics that have been shown to modulate the vagus nerve. Examples of prebiotic-rich foods include onions, garlic, bananas, and whole grains.

- **Timing and Dosage:** Optimal timing and dosage of probiotics can also affect their influence on the vagus nerve. It is recommended to take probiotics on an empty stomach or with a meal that contains some fats, as this can enhance their survival and colonization in the gut. The dosage may vary depending on the specific strain and individual needs, so it is advisable to consult with a healthcare professional for personalized recommendations.

- **Combination with Other Therapies:** The effects of probiotics on the vagus nerve can be further enhanced when combined with other therapies that promote vagal activity. These may include techniques such as deep breathing exercises, meditation, and acupuncture. Combining these techniques with probiotics may create a synergistic effect and improve overall vagus nerve function.

In conclusion, probiotics have the potential to modulate the activity of the vagus nerve through various mechanisms. By improving the balance of gut microbiota, enhancing gut barrier function, regulating inflammation, and influencing neurotransmitter production, probiotics can indirectly affect the vagus nerve and promote overall health. However, further research is needed to fully understand the specific mechanisms through which probiotics interact with the vagus nerve and to determine the most effective ways to optimize their benefits.

NOTE: *This response is for informational purposes only and should not be considered medical advice. It is important to consult with a healthcare professional before starting any new treatment or supplements.*

14. Humming: Humming or making low-pitched sounds can activate the vagus nerve. The vibrations produced during humming stimulate the nerves, helping to relax the body and reduce stress.

The humming of the vagus nerve, also known as vagus nerve stimulation or vagal humming, is a technique that involves producing a continuous, low-pitched vocalization with the mouth closed. This technique has been found to stimulate the vagus nerve, which is the longest cranial nerve in the body and plays a crucial role in the parasympathetic nervous system's regulation of relaxation, digestion, and overall well-being.

Here's a detailed explanation of how humming can positively impact the vagus nerve:

- **Stimulating the vagus nerve:** The vagus nerve is connected to various muscles in the body, including those involved in vocalization. When you hum, you engage and activate the muscles in the back of your throat, which are connected to the vagus nerve. This stimulation of the vagus nerve can have positive effects on heart rate, blood pressure, digestion, and overall relaxation.

- **Relaxation response:** Humming triggers the parasympathetic nervous system's "rest and digest" response, which is controlled by the vagus nerve. This response helps to counteract the "fight or flight" stress response and promotes relaxation, calmness, and a sense of well-being. By humming, you can activate this relaxation response and reduce stress and anxiety.

- **Heart rate variability:** Humming has been found to increase heart rate variability (HRV), which is the variation in time between successive heartbeats. Higher HRV is associated with better cardiovascular health and increased vagal tone, indicating a healthier functioning of the vagus nerve. Humming helps regulate heart rate variability and supports overall heart health.

- **Improved digestion:** The vagus nerve plays a crucial role in the digestive process, controlling the secretion of digestive enzymes, stomach acid production, and the rhythmic contractions of the digestive system. By stimulating the vagus nerve through humming, you can enhance these functions and promote better digestion and nutrient absorption.

- **Enhanced mood and well-being:** The vagus nerve is involved in the regulation of various neurotransmitters, including serotonin and dopamine, which are associated with mood regulation. Stimulating the vagus nerve through humming can help increase the release of these neurotransmitters, leading to improved mood, decreased symptoms of depression, and enhanced overall well-being.

To incorporate humming for vagus nerve stimulation into your routine, follow these steps:

- Find a peaceful and agreeable space where you can sit or rest serenely.

- Close your eyes and take a few deep breaths to relax your body and mind.

- Close your mouth and gently hum with your lips lightly pressed together. Aim for a low-pitched and continuous humming sound.

- Focus on the vibrations you feel in your throat and chest as you hum. Visualize the sound and vibrations positively affecting your vagus nerve and promoting relaxation and well-being.

- Continue humming for a few minutes, allowing yourself to fully engage in the experience.

- After you finish humming, take a moment to stay still and observe any changes in your body, such as increased relaxation, reduced tension, or a sense of calmness.

By incorporating regular humming sessions into your routine, you can stimulate and activate the vagus nerve, leading to numerous benefits for your physical and mental health.

Note: *It's important to note that while humming can be a helpful practice for vagus nerve stimulation and relaxation, it should not replace any medical treatments or therapies prescribed by healthcare professionals. If you have any specific health concerns or conditions, it's always advisable to consult with a healthcare provider before incorporating new practices into your routine.*

15. Positive Affirmations: Repeating positive affirmations or engaging in self-affirmation exercises can activate the vagus nerve by promoting feelings of self-worth and emotional well-being.

Positive affirmations are statements or phrases that we repeat to ourselves to help shift our mindset, promote healing, and improve overall mental and physical health. When it comes to the vagus nerve, positive affirmations can be particularly helpful in activating and promoting its health and functionality.

Here are some ways in which positive affirmations can have a positive impact on the vagus nerve:

- **Stress reduction:** Chronic stress can have a detrimental effect on the vagus nerve, leading to decreased vagal tone and potential health problems. By incorporating positive affirmations into our daily routine, we can lower stress levels and promote better vagal tone. Confirmations, for example, "I'm quiet and settled," "I discharge pressure and strain from my body and psyche," or "I'm in charge of my reaction to stretch" can help activate the vagus nerve's relaxation response.

- **Improved digestion:** The vagus nerve plays a significant role in digestion by regulating the movement of food through the digestive tract, stimulating digestive enzymes, and promoting nutrient absorption. Positive affirmations that focus on healthy digestion, such as "I nourish my body with healthy food," "My digestive system is strong and efficient," or "I embrace and trust the regular course of assimilation," can help initiate and back the vagus nerve's stomach related capabilities.

- **Enhanced heart health:** The vagus nerve has a direct impact on heart rate variability, which is an indicator of the heart's ability to adapt to changing physiological demands. Positive affirmations that promote cardiovascular health, such as "My heart beats in perfect harmony," "I am grateful for my healthy heart," or "I am in tune with my heart's wisdom," can activate the vagus nerve and improve heart rate variability, leading to better heart health.

- **Emotional regulation:** The vagus nerve is closely linked to our emotional well-being and plays a role in regulating our emotional responses. Positive affirmations that focus on emotional balance and regulation, such as "I am in control of my emotions," "I embrace and release my emotions with love," or "I create a peaceful and emotionally balanced environment within me," can activate the vagus nerve and promote emotional resilience.

- **Better immune function:** The vagus nerve also influences the immune system and helps regulate the body's inflammatory response. Positive affirmations that support a healthy immune system, such as "I am strong and resilient," "I am protected and supported by my immune system," or "I trust in my body's ability to heal itself," can activate the vagus nerve and enhance immune function.

- **Improved overall well-being:** By activating the vagus nerve through positive affirmations, we can experience an overall sense of well-being. Affirmations that promote self-love, self-acceptance, and inner peace, such as "I love and accept myself unconditionally," "I am deserving of love and happiness," or "I'm associated with the heavenly insight inside me," can initiate the vagus nerve and advance a condition of by and large prosperity, prompting worked on physical, mental, and profound well-being.

NOTE: *It is important to note that while positive affirmations can be a valuable tool in promoting the health and functionality of the vagus nerve, they should not replace medical treatment or professional guidance. If you are experiencing any specific health concerns, it is always advisable to consult with a healthcare professional.*

CHAPTER FOUR

4.0. The Role of Nutrition in Vagus Nerve Health

It plays a vital role in regulating various bodily functions, including digestion, heart rate, respiration, and autonomic control. Nutrition has a significant impact on vagus nerve health due to the following reasons:

- **Nerve function and repair:** The vagus nerve relies on specific nutrients to maintain its structural integrity and proper functioning. Adequate amounts of vitamins, minerals, and antioxidants are essential for nerve cell formation, regeneration, and repair. Deficiencies in essential nutrients like vitamin B12, vitamin D, magnesium, and omega-3 fatty acids can lead to nerve damage, inflammation, and decreased vagus nerve health.

- **Neurotransmitter production:** The vagus nerve relies on a delicate balance of neurotransmitters for proper communication between nerve cells and target organs. Nutrition plays a key role in the production, release, and regulation of these neurotransmitters. For instance, the amino acids tryptophan and tyrosine obtained from protein-rich foods are precursors for producing neurotransmitters like serotonin, dopamine, and norepinephrine, which are essential for maintaining vagus nerve function.

- **Gut-brain axis:** The vagus nerve is intricately connected to the enteric nervous system (ENS), often referred to as the "second brain." The ENS consists of a network of neurons lining the gastrointestinal tract, which communicates bidirectionally with the central nervous system, including the vagus nerve. Nutrition plays a critical role in the health of the gut microbiota, which in turn influences the communication between the gut and the brain through the vagus nerve. A healthy and diverse microbiota, achieved through a balanced and varied diet, promotes optimal vagus nerve function and overall well-being.

- **Inflammation and oxidative stress:** Chronic inflammation and oxidative stress can negatively affect vagus nerve health. Nutrition plays a crucial role in reducing inflammation and oxidative stress by providing antioxidants and promoting an anti-inflammatory environment. Diets high in fruits, vegetables, and whole grains are rich in antioxidants, which protect nerve cells from damage caused by harmful free radicals. Additionally, omega-3 fatty acids found in fatty fish, flaxseed, and walnuts have anti-inflammatory properties that can support vagus nerve health.

- **Blood glucose regulation:** Unstable blood glucose levels can impact the function of the vagus nerve. Eating a balanced diet that includes complex carbohydrates, healthy fats, and protein can help maintain stable blood sugar levels throughout the day. This, in turn, supports the optimal functioning of the vagus nerve, which helps regulate glucose metabolism and insulin sensitivity.

- **Stress modulation:** The vagus nerve plays a crucial role in the body's stress response by activating the relaxation response and reducing the release of stress hormones. Nutrients like magnesium, B vitamins, and omega-3 fatty acids have been shown to support healthy stress responses and promote a calm and balanced nervous system, indirectly supporting vagus nerve health.

In summary, nutrition plays a fundamental role in maintaining and supporting vagus nerve health. A balanced and nutrient-rich diet provides the necessary building blocks for nerve cell formation, repair, and function. It also supports gut-brain communication and helps reduce inflammation, oxidative stress, and blood sugar imbalances that can negatively impact the vagus nerve. By prioritizing a wholesome diet, individuals can support optimal vagus nerve function and overall well-being.

NOTE: *The data given here is too instructive and ought not to be considered as clinical counsel. It is constantly prescribed to talk with a medical care professional for customized direction and proposals regarding nourishment and well-being.*

4.1 Foods That Promote Vagus Nerve Activation

Certain foods can support vagus nerve activation and enhance its function. These foods either stimulate the production of neurotransmitters or provide nutrients that support nerve health.

Here are some examples:

- **Omega-3 fatty acids:** Foods rich in omega-3 fatty acids, such as fatty fish (salmon, mackerel, sardines), flaxseeds, chia seeds, and walnuts, can support vagus nerve health. Omega-3 fatty acids have anti-inflammatory properties, which can help reduce inflammation and promote optimal nerve function.

- **Prebiotic and probiotic-rich foods:** Prebiotics are types of dietary fiber that feed the beneficial gut bacteria, while probiotics are live bacteria that provide health benefits. Both prebiotics and probiotics promote a healthy gut microbiome, which supports the communication between the gut and the brain through the vagus nerve. Examples of prebiotic-rich foods include onions, garlic, asparagus, bananas, and artichokes. Probiotic-rich food sources incorporate yogurt, kefir, sauerkraut, kimchi, and fermented tea.

- **Antioxidant-rich foods:** Antioxidants help protect against oxidative stress and reduce inflammation, supporting the overall health of the vagus nerve. Foods high in antioxidants include fruits (berries, cherries, citrus fruits), vegetables (spinach, kale, bell peppers), nuts (almonds, walnuts), and green tea.

- **Magnesium-rich foods:** Magnesium plays a crucial role in nerve function and helps regulate neurotransmitters. Foods rich in magnesium include leafy green vegetables (spinach, kale, Swiss chard), legumes, nuts, seeds, and whole grains.

- **B vitamins:** B vitamins, especially vitamins B6, B12, and folate, are essential for nerve health and neurotransmitter synthesis. Foods rich in B vitamins include lean meats, poultry, fish, eggs, dairy products, leafy green vegetables, legumes, fortified cereals, and nutritional yeast.

- **Tryptophan-rich foods:** Tryptophan is an essential amino acid that serves as a precursor to serotonin, an important neurotransmitter involved in mood regulation and stress management. Foods rich in tryptophan include turkey, chicken, eggs, nuts, seeds, and tofu.

- **Dark chocolate:** Dark chocolate contains flavonoids that have been shown to stimulate the release of nitric oxide, which in turn supports vagus nerve function. Opt for dark chocolate with a high percentage of cacao (70% or higher) and minimal added sugars.

- **Herbal teas:** Certain herbal teas, such as chamomile, lavender, and lemon balm, have calming properties that can stimulate vagus nerve activity and promote relaxation.

NOTE: It is important to note that while these foods can support vagus nerve activation, they should be part of a balanced and varied diet. It is always recommended to consult with a healthcare professional or registered dietitian for personalized advice and guidance on incorporating these foods into your diet.

4.2. Probiotics and Gut Health

The gut and the vagus nerve have a close and bidirectional relationship, known as the gut-brain axis. The gut microbiota, which is a collection of trillions of bacteria residing in our gastrointestinal tract, plays a vital role in this relationship. Probiotics, frequently alluded to as "great microbes," are live microorganisms that present medical advantages when consumed in sufficient sums.

Here's how probiotics and gut health can influence the vagus nerve:

- **Modulation of neurotransmitters:** The gut microbiota can produce and influence the production of neurotransmitters, such as serotonin, dopamine, and gamma-aminobutyric acid (GABA). These neurotransmitters play a critical part in managing temperament, tension, and stress reactions. The vagus nerve, as the main communication pathway between the gut and the brain, is involved in transmitting these signals. Probiotics can modulate the production and availability of these neurotransmitters, which can influence vagus nerve activity and overall brain function.

- **Regulation of inflammation:** The gut microbiota plays a significant role in regulating immune responses and inflammation. Dysbiosis, an imbalance in the gut microbiota characterized by an overgrowth of harmful bacteria and a decrease in beneficial bacteria, can lead to chronic inflammation. In turn, this inflammation can negatively impact vagus nerve function. Probiotics help restore a healthy balance of gut bacteria, reducing inflammation and promoting vagus nerve health.

- **Production of short-chain fatty acids (SCFAs):** Probiotics in the gut microbiota ferment dietary fibers and produce SCFAs, such as butyrate, acetate, and propionate. SCFAs have protective effects on the gut barrier, regulate immune responses, and play a role in modulating the vagus nerve activity. Butyrate, in particular, has been shown to enhance the function of the vagus nerve and improve gut-brain communication.

- **Improvement of gut barrier function:** The gut barrier serves as a protective barrier between the gut and the bloodstream. A compromised gut barrier, often referred to as "leaky gut," can lead to the entry of harmful bacteria and toxins into the bloodstream, triggering immune responses and inflammation. Probiotics help support the integrity of the gut barrier, preventing permeability and maintaining a healthy gut-brain axis. This directly affects the communication between the gut and the vagus nerve.

- **Reduction of oxidative stress:** Oxidative stress occurs when there is an imbalance between antioxidants and harmful free radicals in the body. The gut microbiota, when unbalanced, can contribute to oxidative stress. Probiotics have been shown to reduce oxidative stress and support antioxidant defenses. By reducing oxidative stress, probiotics indirectly support vagus nerve health.

- **Regulation of stress response:** Chronic stress can negatively impact the gut microbiota and vagus nerve function. Probiotics have been found to regulate the body's stress response, reducing the release of stress hormones and promoting a calmer nervous system. This can support the optimal functioning of the vagus nerve and its role in stress modulation.

NOTE: It is worth noting that more research is needed to fully understand the complex interactions between the gut microbiota, probiotics, and the vagus nerve. However, the existing evidence suggests that a healthy gut microbiota supported by probiotics can positively influence vagus nerve function and overall gut-brain communication. Incorporating probiotic-rich foods (such as yogurt, kefir, and fermented vegetables) or taking probiotic supplements may help support vagus nerve health, but it is essential to consult with a healthcare professional for personalized advice.

4.3. Anti-inflammatory Diet for Vagus Nerve Support

The vagus nerve is an essential part of the body's relaxation response and plays a crucial role in regulating inflammation. An anti-inflammatory diet can be beneficial for supporting the vagus nerve and reducing inflammation in the body.

Here is a detailed explanation of the anti-inflammatory diet for vagus nerve support:

- **Focus on Whole Foods:** The foundation of the anti-inflammatory diet is whole, unprocessed foods. This incorporates organic products, vegetables, entire grains, vegetables, nuts, and seeds. These foods are rich in fiber, antioxidants, vitamins, and minerals, which help reduce inflammation and support overall health.

- **Omega-3 Fatty Acids:** Incorporating foods rich in omega-3 fatty acids is essential for reducing inflammation. Good sources include fatty fish like salmon, mackerel, and sardines; chia seeds, flaxseeds, and walnuts. Omega-3 fatty acids help balance the production of certain chemicals in the body that promote inflammation.

- **Healthy Fats:** Including healthy fats in the diet is crucial as they support the production of anti-inflammatory compounds. Focus on sources like extra virgin olive oil, avocados, coconut oil, and nuts. These fats also help with the absorption of fat-soluble vitamins and provide sustained energy.

- **Turmeric and Ginger:** Turmeric and ginger are powerful anti-inflammatory spices. They contain curcumin and gingerol, respectively, which have been shown to reduce inflammation in the body. Including these spices in your meals or taking them as supplements can help support the vagus nerve and reduce inflammation.

- **Colorful Fruits and Vegetables:** Incorporating a variety of colorful fruits and vegetables into your diet provides a wide range of antioxidants, phytochemicals, and vitamins that have anti-inflammatory effects. Aim for a diverse range of fruits and vegetables, including leafy greens, berries, tomatoes, broccoli, and peppers.

- **Avoid Trigger Foods:** Some foods may trigger inflammation in the body for individuals. Common culprits include processed foods, refined sugars, trans fats, and excessive intake of alcohol and caffeine. Pay attention to your body's response to certain foods and try to eliminate or limit those that may cause inflammation.

- **Probiotics:** Probiotics are beneficial bacteria that support gut health, which in turn can help reduce inflammation in the body. Include fermented foods like yogurt, kefir, sauerkraut, kimchi, and kombucha in your diet to promote a healthy gut microbiome.

- **Hydration:** Staying hydrated is essential for overall health and supporting the vagus nerve. Drink plenty of water throughout the day to stay hydrated and help flush out toxins from the body.

- **Mindful Eating:** Practicing mindful eating can also support the vagus nerve and reduce inflammation. Slow down while eating, chew your food thoroughly, and pay attention to the taste, texture, and sensation of each bite. This helps activate the parasympathetic nervous system, which is responsible for the body's relaxation response and vagus nerve activation.

- **Stress Management:** Chronic stress can contribute to inflammation in the body. Incorporate stress management techniques like meditation, deep breathing exercises, yoga, and regular exercise into your daily routine. These practices help activate the vagus nerve and promote relaxation, reducing inflammation.

NOTE: *It's important to note that individual dietary needs may vary, and consulting with a healthcare professional or registered dietitian can help create a personalized anti-inflammatory diet plan for vagus nerve support.*

Overall, the anti-inflammatory diet for vagus nerve support focuses on consuming whole, unprocessed foods, incorporating omega-3 fatty acids and healthy fats, including turmeric and ginger, consuming colorful fruits and vegetables, avoiding trigger foods, consuming probiotics, staying hydrated, practicing mindful eating, and managing stress. Following this diet can help support the vagus nerve and reduce inflammation in the body, promoting overall health and well-being.

Chapter Five

5.0. Lifestyle Changes for Vagus Nerve Stimulation

Several lifestyle changes can support and stimulate the vagus nerve, which is responsible for the body's relaxation response and overall well-being.

Here is a detailed explanation of these lifestyle changes for vagus nerve stimulation:

- **Deep Breathing Exercises:** Deep breathing exercises, such as diaphragmatic breathing or belly breathing, can activate the vagus nerve and promote relaxation. This involves taking slow, deep breaths, filling the belly with air, and exhaling slowly. It helps activate the parasympathetic nervous system and reduces stress and anxiety.

- **Meditation:** Regular meditation practice has been shown to stimulate the vagus nerve and increase its activity. Care contemplation, for instance, includes concentrating on the current second without judgment. This can help reduce stress and anxiety, promote relaxation, and support vagus nerve function.

- **Yoga:** Yoga combines physical movements, breathwork, and meditation, making it an ideal practice for vagus nerve stimulation. Certain yoga poses, such as Bridge Pose, Fish Pose, and Shoulder Stand, specifically target the throat and neck area, where the vagus nerve is located. Regular yoga practice can improve overall vagal tone, promoting relaxation and reducing inflammation.

- **Cold Exposure:** Cold exposure, such as cold showers or cold water immersion, can activate the vagus nerve. Cold stimulates the body's sympathetic nervous system response, but when the body adapts to the cold, the parasympathetic nervous system, which is regulated by the vagus nerve, kicks in, promoting relaxation. Begin with short openings to cold and continuously increment the length and force over the long haul.

- **Regular Exercise:** Engaging in regular physical exercise, such as aerobic activities or strength training, can stimulate the vagus nerve. Exercise has been shown to increase heart rate variability, which is an indicator of vagal tone. Aim for at least 30 minutes of moderate-intensity exercise most days of the week to support vagus nerve function.

- **Social Connections:** Building and maintaining strong social connections is crucial for vagus nerve stimulation. Positive social interactions, such as spending time with loved ones, participating in group activities, or engaging in meaningful conversations, activate the vagus nerve and promote feelings of well-being and relaxation.

- **Laughter:** Laughter has been shown to stimulate the vagus nerve and promote relaxation. Engage in activities that make you laugh, such as watching funny videos, spending time with funny friends, or participating in laughter yoga classes. This can help reduce stress, boost mood, and support vagus nerve function.

- **Mindfulness and Stress Reduction:** Practicing mindfulness and stress reduction techniques can support vagus nerve stimulation. Engage in activities such as journaling, listening to calming music, spending time in nature, taking warm baths, or engaging in hobbies that bring joy and relaxation. These activities help reduce stress and activate the vagus nerve.

- **Regular Sleep Routine:** Getting sufficient and quality sleep is vital for vagus nerve stimulation and overall health. Hold back nothing long periods of continuous rest every evening and lay out a steady rest schedule. Create a relaxing bedtime routine, avoid stimulating substances like caffeine and electronics before bed, and create a comfortable sleep environment to support vagus nerve function.

- **Healthy Diet:** Following a healthy diet, such as the anti-inflammatory diet mentioned earlier, supports vagus nerve stimulation. Consuming whole, unprocessed foods, incorporating omega-3 fatty acids, and avoiding trigger foods can help reduce inflammation and support vagus nerve health.

NOTE: *It's important to note that these lifestyle changes may have different effects on individuals, and it's recommended to consult with a healthcare* *professional for personalized guidance and support in stimulating the vagus nerve.*

In summary, lifestyle changes for vagus nerve stimulation include deep breathing exercises, meditation, yoga, cold exposure, regular exercise, social connections, laughter, mindfulness and stress reduction techniques, a regular sleep routine, and maintaining a healthy diet. These lifestyle changes can help activate the vagus nerve, promote relaxation, reduce stress, and support overall well-being.

5.1. Stress Reduction Techniques

Stress reduction techniques can be highly beneficial for stimulating and supporting the vagus nerve. The vagus nerve is involved in the body's relaxation response, and reducing stress can help activate this nerve and promote a sense of calm and well-being.

Here are some stress reduction techniques that specifically target the vagus nerve:

- **Deep Breathing:** Deep breathing exercises, such as diaphragmatic breathing or belly breathing, are simple yet effective techniques for vagus nerve stimulation. By taking slow, deep breaths and filling the belly with air, you activate the diaphragm, which in turn stimulates the vagus nerve and promotes relaxation. Aim to breathe in deeply for a count of four, hold the breath for a count of four, and exhale slowly for a count of four.

- **Meditation:** Mindfulness meditation and other forms of meditation have been shown to activate the vagus nerve and reduce stress. During meditation, focus your attention on the present moment, observing your thoughts and sensations without judgment. This helps quiet the mind, reduce anxiety, and promote overall relaxation.

- **Moderate Muscle Unwinding:** Moderate muscle unwinding includes straining and afterward delivering different muscle bunches in the body. By deliberately tensing and then fully relaxing each muscle group, you can release tension and promote relaxation throughout the body. This technique helps activate the vagus nerve and reduce stress.

- **Yoga:** Yoga combines physical postures, breath control, and meditation, making it a comprehensive stress reduction technique that stimulates the vagus nerve. Certain yoga poses, such as forward folds, gentle twists, and restorative poses, specifically target the throat and neck area where the vagus nerve is located. Regular practice of yoga can help reduce stress, promote relaxation, and support vagus nerve function.

- **Directed Symbolism:** Directed symbolism includes imagining tranquil scenes or circumstances. By using your imagination to create a mental image of a relaxing place, such as a beach or a forest, you can activate the vagus nerve and reduce stress. Guided imagery can be done with the help of audio recordings or by following a script, guiding your own imagination.

- **Laughter Therapy:** Laughter has been shown to stimulate the vagus nerve and promote relaxation. Engaging in activities that make you laugh, such as watching funny videos, spending time with humorous friends, or participating in laughter yoga classes, can help reduce stress and activate the vagus nerve.

- **Massage Therapy:** Massage therapy can help relax tense muscles, reduce stress, and stimulate the vagus nerve. The physical manipulation and pressure applied during a massage can promote relaxation and activate the parasympathetic nervous system, which is regulated by the vagus nerve.

- **Mindfulness-Based Stress Reduction (MBSR):** MBSR is a structured program that combines mindfulness meditation, body awareness, and yoga. It is specifically designed to reduce stress and promote well-being. By participating in MBSR programs, individuals can learn various techniques that stimulate the vagus nerve, reduce stress, and enhance resilience.

- **Nature Therapy:** Spending time in nature has been shown to reduce stress levels and activate the vagus nerve. Engage in outdoor activities such as walking in the park, hiking, gardening, or simply sitting in a natural environment. The calming sights, sounds, and smells of nature can promote relaxation and vagus nerve stimulation.

- **Gratitude Practice:** Cultivating a practice of gratitude involves expressing appreciation for the positive aspects of life. This practice has been shown to reduce stress and activate the vagus nerve. Take a few moments each day to acknowledge and reflect on the things you are grateful for. This can be done through journaling or sharing gratitude with others.

NOTE: *Remember that individual preferences and responses may vary, and it's important to explore different stress reduction techniques to find what works best for you. Incorporating these stress reduction techniques into your daily routine can help stimulate and support the vagus nerve, reduce stress, and promote overall well-being. If you have any specific health concerns or conditions, it's important to consult with a healthcare professional for personalized guidance and support.*

5.2 Sleep Hygiene and Vagus Nerve Health

Sleep hygiene refers to a set of practices and habits that help individuals establish a healthy sleep routine and promote better quality sleep. These practices contribute to overall well-being and can improve physical and mental health. On the other hand, the vagus nerve is the longest cranial nerve in the body, which plays a crucial role in regulating various bodily functions, including digestion, heart rate, inflammation, and relaxation. Maintaining a healthy vagus nerve can lead to improved overall health and well-being.

Sleep Hygiene:

- **Consistent bedtime routine:** Establishing a consistent sleep schedule by going to bed and waking up at the same time every day, even on weekends, helps regulate the body's internal clock.

- **Create a sleep-friendly environment:** Make sure the bedroom is cool, quiet, and dark, as these conditions promote better sleep. Use earplugs, eye masks, or white noise machines if needed.

- **Limit exposure to electronic devices:** The blue light emitted from electronic devices can interfere with natural sleep patterns. Avoid using devices such as phones, tablets, or computers for at least an hour before bed.

- **Avoid stimulants:** Limit the intake of caffeine, nicotine, and excessive alcohol, especially close to bedtime. These substances can interfere with sleep, causing restlessness or fragmented sleep.

- **Normal activity:** Participating in standard actual work during the day can advance better rest around evening time. Be that as it may, keep away from vivacious activity near sleep time, as it might obstruct rest.

- **Manage stress:** Stress and anxiety can disrupt sleep. Practicing relaxation techniques such as deep breathing, meditation, or listening to calming music can help reduce stress levels and promote better sleep.

- **Avoid napping:** If possible, avoid taking long or late afternoon naps, as they may interfere with nighttime sleep. If a nap is necessary, limit it to a short duration and before 3 pm.

- **Avoid heavy meals and liquids before bed:** Eating a heavy meal or consuming excessive fluids close to bedtime may disrupt sleep due to digestion or bathroom trips. It's recommended to have a light snack if necessary.

- **Create a sleep-friendly bedtime routine:** Implementing activities such as reading, taking a warm bath, or practicing gentle stretching before bed can signal the body that it's time to relax and prepare for sleep.

NOTE: *It's important to note that while practicing good sleep hygiene and promoting vagus nerve health can have significant benefits, individual experiences may vary. It's always best to consult with a healthcare professional for personalized advice and guidance on maintaining optimal sleep and nerve health.*

5.3 Exercise and Physical Activity

Engaging in exercise and physical activity can have a positive impact on vagal tone, which is the measure of the vagus nerve's activity and function.

Here is an explanation of how exercise and physical activity can affect the vagus nerve:

- **Increase heart rate variability (HRV):** HRV is the variation in the time interval between heartbeats. A higher HRV indicates a healthier heart and a better vagal tone. Regular aerobic exercise and cardiovascular workouts have been shown to increase HRV, indicating increased vagal activity and improved vagus nerve function.

- **Promote relaxation and reduce stress:** Engaging in physical activity triggers the release of endorphins, often referred to as "feel-good" hormones. These endorphins help reduce stress levels and promote relaxation, activating the parasympathetic nervous system, which is regulated by the vagus nerve. This can lead to increased vagal tone and improved vagus nerve health.

- **Enhance respiratory function:** Exercise that involves deep breathing, such as yoga or tai chi, can stimulate the vagus nerve and improve respiratory function. Deep breathing exercises activate the relaxation response and engage the diaphragm, helping to regulate and strengthen the vagus nerve.

- **Improve gut health:** The vagus nerve plays a crucial role in the gut-brain connection, influencing digestion and gut health. Regular exercise has been shown to improve gut motility, reduce the risk of gastrointestinal disorders, and enhance overall gut health. The vagus nerve is involved in these processes, and exercise can stimulate its activity, leading to improved gut function.

- **Reduce inflammation:** Inflammation in the body is associated with various health conditions. The vagus nerve has anti-inflammatory properties, and exercising regularly can enhance its function. Physical activity helps regulate the immune system, reducing inflammation and promoting overall health.

- **Enhance mood and mental well-being:** Engaging in exercise and physical activity has been linked to improved mood and mental well-being. Exercise releases endorphins and other chemicals that elevate mood and reduce symptoms of depression and anxiety. These positive effects on mental health can be attributed, at least in part, to the vagus nerve, as it is involved in regulating emotions and stress responses.

- **Improve brain function:** The vagus nerve has connections to various regions of the brain, including those involved in learning, memory, and cognitive function. Regular exercise has been shown to enhance brain health and improve cognitive function.

The increased blood flow and oxygenation to the brain, stimulated by exercise, can positively impact the vagus nerve and its function.

NOTE: *It's important to note that the relationship between exercise and the vagus nerve is complex, and individual responses may vary. The type, duration, and intensity of exercise can influence the effects on vagal tone and overall vagus nerve health. Additionally, it's always recommended to consult with a healthcare professional before starting or changing an exercise routine, especially if you have any underlying health conditions or concerns.*

5.4 Mindfulness Practices for Vagus Nerve Stimulation

Mindfulness practices can help stimulate and activate the vagus nerve, promoting relaxation, reducing stress, and improving overall well-being. By engaging in these practices, you can enhance vagal tone and support the optimal function of the vagus nerve.

Here are some mindfulness practices that can stimulate the vagus nerve:

1. Deep Breathing: Deep breathing exercises that focus on prolonging the exhale activate the relaxation response and stimulate the vagus nerve. One simple technique is diaphragmatic breathing, where you inhale deeply through your nose, allowing your belly to expand, and exhale fully through your mouth, feeling your belly contract. Aim for slow, deep, and controlled breaths.

2. Body Scan Meditation: This mindfulness practice involves systematically scanning your body from head to toe, bringing attention to each area and noticing any sensations or tension. As you bring awareness to different body parts, consciously relaxing and releasing tension can activate the vagus nerve and promote relaxation.

3. Loving-Kindness Meditation: Also known as Metta meditation, this practice involves cultivating feelings of compassion, love, and kindness towards oneself and others. By generating positive feelings and focusing on goodwill, this meditation can activate the vagus nerve and promote a sense of connection and well-being.

4. Mindful Eating: Paying close attention to the sensations, tastes, and smells while eating can stimulate the vagus nerve and promote better digestion. Chew slowly, savor each bite, and be fully present in the experience of eating.

5. Progressive Muscle Relaxation: This technique involves systematically tensing and then relaxing different muscle groups in the body, promoting physical and mental relaxation. By consciously releasing tension and promoting muscle relaxation, you can activate the vagus nerve and enhance its function.

6. Mindful Walking or Movement: Engaging in mindful walking or movement practices such as yoga, tai chi, or qigong can stimulate the vagus nerve. The combination of movement, breath awareness, and mindfulness can induce a relaxed state, activate the parasympathetic nervous system, and enhance vagal tone.

7. Mindful Listening: Focusing intentionally on sounds in your environment can be a way to enhance mindfulness and stimulate the vagus nerve. Pay attention to the different sounds around you, without judgment or analysis. This practice can help bring you into the present moment, enhancing relaxation and stress reduction.

8. Mindfulness-Based Stress Reduction (MBSR): MBSR is an evidence-based program that combines mindfulness meditation, body awareness, and yoga. It aims to help individuals develop a greater awareness of their thoughts, emotions, and bodily sensations. By practicing MBSR, you can enhance vagal tone and promote overall well-being.

9. Mindful Breathing Exercises: In addition to deep breathing, different breathing exercises can specifically stimulate the vagus nerve. For example, alternate nostril breathing involves closing one nostril and inhaling deeply, then closing the other nostril and exhaling fully. This rhythmic breathing pattern can activate the vagus nerve and induce relaxation.

10. Guided Imagery: Guided imagery involves visualizing specific peaceful or calming scenes, such as a serene beach or a tranquil forest. By immersing yourself in these mental images, you can stimulate the vagus nerve, promote relaxation, and reduce stress.

NOTE: *It's important to note that consistency and regular practice are key to experiencing the benefits* *of mindfulness practices for vagus nerve stimulation. Find the techniques that resonate with you and incorporate them into your daily routine. It's also beneficial to seek guidance from a qualified mindfulness instructor or therapist, especially if you are new to these practices or have specific mental health concerns.*

Additionally, it's important to remember that the effectiveness of mindfulness practices for vagus nerve stimulation may vary from person to person. Different individuals may respond differently to various techniques, and it may take time to find the practices that work best for you. It's also crucial to approach these practices with an open mind and gentle self-compassion, allowing yourself to explore and discover what feels most beneficial for your mind and body.

Chapter Six

6.0. Vagus Nerve and Mental Health

In recent years, scientific research has shown a strong connection between the vagus nerve and mental health. The vagus nerve plays a crucial role in the regulation of the parasympathetic nervous system, which is involved in the body's rest and digestion response. This system works in opposition to the sympathetic nervous system, responsible for the fight-or-flight response.

Stimulation of the vagus nerve has been found to reduce anxiety and stress and improve mood and overall well-being. One of the ways the vagus nerve affects mental health is through its influence on the release of neurotransmitters such as serotonin and dopamine, which are responsible for mood regulation. Studies have shown that vagus nerve stimulation increases the production of these "feel-good" neurotransmitters, leading to an improvement in symptoms of depression and anxiety.

The vagus nerve also has a direct impact on the stress response. When activated, it helps to calm down the nervous system and reduce the release of stress hormones, such as cortisol and adrenaline. This helps to alleviate feelings of anxiety and promotes a sense of relaxation and calmness.

Additionally, the vagus nerve is closely connected to the gut-brain axis, which refers to the bidirectional communication between the central nervous system (CNS) and the gastrointestinal system. The stomach is frequently alluded to as the "second mind" because of its broad organization of neurons and neurotransmitters. The vagus nerve plays a critical role in transmitting signals between the gut and the brain, influencing digestion, nutrient absorption, and overall gut health.

Emerging research has implicated disturbances in the gut-brain axis in various mental health conditions, including depression, anxiety, and even neurodevelopmental disorders like autism. It is believed that imbalances in the gut microbiota (the trillions of bacteria residing in the gut) can affect the vagus nerve and consequently impact mental health. Disruptions in the vagus nerve's signaling can lead to inflammation, which has been linked to depression and other mood disorders.

There are several techniques to stimulate the vagus nerve and improve mental health.

One common method is called vagus nerve stimulation (VNS), which involves a medical device implanted in the body that delivers electrical impulses to the vagus nerve. VNS has been approved by the FDA as a treatment for epilepsy and treatment-resistant depression. It has also shown promise in reducing symptoms of anxiety disorders and enhancing overall well-being.

Another method to stimulate the vagus nerve is through deep breathing exercises. Slow, deep breaths activate the parasympathetic nervous system and stimulate the vagus nerve, leading to a relaxation response. Techniques such as diaphragmatic breathing, alternate nostril breathing, and paced breathing can be effective in promoting vagal tone and reducing anxiety.

Physical exercise has also been shown to stimulate the vagus nerve. Regular aerobic exercise has been linked to increased vagal tone, which boosts mental health and resilience to stress. Activities like running, swimming, and cycling can positively impact vagus nerve function.

Additionally, certain lifestyle changes can promote vagus nerve health and improve mental well-being. These include stress management techniques such as meditation, yoga, and mindfulness exercises. Getting enough sleep, maintaining a healthy diet rich in omega-3 fatty acids, and reducing exposure to toxins and pollutants can also support the health of the vagus nerve and overall mental wellness.

In summary, the vagus nerve plays a significant role in mental health. Its connection to the parasympathetic nervous system, stress response, neurotransmitter release, and gut-brain axis makes it a key player in regulating mood, anxiety, and overall well-being. Stimulating the vagus nerve through various techniques can have a positive impact on mental health, reducing symptoms of depression, anxiety, and stress. Further research into this complex relationship between the vagus nerve and mental health is ongoing, and it holds potential for the development of new interventions and therapies for mental health disorders.

6.1 Anxiety and the Vagus Nerve

Anxiety is a common mental health disorder characterized by excessive worrying, fear, and nervousness. It can cause various physical symptoms, such as a rapid heartbeat, shortness of breath, chest pain, trembling, sweating, and gastrointestinal issues like stomach aches or nausea.

The vagus nerve, otherwise called the 10th cranial nerve, is the longest and most complex nerve in the body. It has multiple branches that connect the brain to various organs, including the heart, lungs, digestive system, and other abdominal organs. The vagus nerve plays a crucial role in regulating several body functions, including heart rate, digestion, respiration, and even the release of certain hormones.

One of the main functions of the vagus nerve is its role in the body's stress response system. When we experience a stressful situation or perceive a threat, the body activates the sympathetic nervous system, which triggers the release of stress hormones like cortisol and adrenaline. Simultaneously, the parasympathetic nervous system, which the vagus nerve is a part of, works to counterbalance the stress response and restore the body to a state of relaxation.

However, in individuals with anxiety disorders, this regulation process can be dysregulated, leading to an overactive sympathetic nervous system and an underactive parasympathetic nervous system. This imbalance can cause an exaggerated stress response and difficulty in returning to a state of relaxation after a stressful event.

The vagus nerve plays a significant role in regulating various physical symptoms commonly associated with anxiety. For example:

- **Heart Rate:** The vagus nerve helps regulate heart rate by sending signals from the brain to the heart. In individuals with anxiety, the activation of the sympathetic nervous system can cause an increased heart rate (tachycardia) and palpitations. The overactive sympathetic response may to some extent inhibit the action of the vagus nerve, leading to an imbalance in heart rate regulation.

- **Digestion:** The vagus nerve also influences digestion by controlling the contractions of the esophagus, stomach, and intestines. Anxiety can impact the functioning of the gastrointestinal system, leading to symptoms such as stomach aches, indigestion, bloating, and even diarrhea. The dysregulation of the vagus nerve's influence on the digestive system may contribute to these symptoms.

- **Respiratory Capability:** The vagus nerve is engaged with controlling the muscles answerable for relaxing.

During moments of heightened anxiety, individuals may experience shallow or rapid breathing, chest tightness, and shortness of breath. These symptoms are influenced by the activation of the sympathetic nervous system and can be further intensified by an imbalance in the regulation of the vagus nerve.

- **Emotional Regulation:** The vagus nerve is also involved in the regulation of emotions and mental health. It has connections to various regions of the brain, including areas responsible for emotional processing and regulation. In individuals with anxiety, the dysregulation of the vagus nerve can impact their emotional states, making it more challenging to regulate anxiety and stress levels.

Understanding the connection between anxiety and the vagus nerve highlights the importance of a comprehensive approach to managing anxiety disorders. Treatment approaches often include a combination of therapy (such as cognitive-behavioral therapy), medications, relaxation techniques, and lifestyle changes to address the dysregulation of the vagus nerve and restore balance to the autonomic nervous system.

6.2. Depression and the Vagus Nerve

Depression is a mental health disorder characterized by persistent feelings of sadness, loss of interest or pleasure in activities, changes in appetite or weight, sleep disturbances, fatigue, difficulty concentrating, and even suicidal thoughts or behaviors. The exact cause of depression is complex and involves a combination of genetic, environmental, and biochemical factors.

Research has suggested a significant association between the vagus nerve and depression. Here are some key points:

Neurotransmitters: The vagus nerve plays a role in regulating the release of neurotransmitters, such as serotonin and norepinephrine, which are crucial for mood regulation. Imbalances in these neurotransmitters are often observed in individuals with depression. The vagus nerve helps stimulate the release of these neurotransmitters and influences their availability in the brain.

- **Inflammation:** The vagus nerve is involved in a process known as the "inflammatory reflex." This reflex helps regulate the body's immune response and inflammation levels. Inflammation has been linked to depression, and the vagus nerve helps regulate the inflammatory response by transmitting signals to reduce inflammation. Dysfunction or impairment of the vagus nerve can disrupt this regulatory process and contribute to increased inflammation, potentially leading to depressive symptoms.

- **HPA Axis:** The vagus nerve also interacts with the hypothalamic-pituitary-adrenal (HPA) axis, which plays a crucial role in the body's stress response. Chronic stress and dysregulation of the HPA axis are common aspects of depression. The vagus nerve helps modulate the HPA axis activity, and dysfunction in the vagal regulation may contribute to an overactive stress response and impair the body's ability to cope with stress, exacerbating depressive symptoms.

- **Heart Rate Variability (HRV):** HRV refers to the variation in time intervals between consecutive heartbeats. It is considered a marker of autonomic nervous system activity, including vagal tone. Reduced HRV has been associated with depression, indicating diminished vagal tone. This suggests that individuals with depression may have decreased vagal activity, which can have negative effects on mood regulation and emotional well-being

- **Gut-Brain Axis:** Emerging research suggests a connection between the gut microbiome and mental health, including depression. The vagus nerve plays a role in the bidirectional communication between the gut and the brain, forming the gut-brain axis. The gut microbiome influences the vagus nerve, and in turn, the vagus nerve influences the gut microbiome. Dysregulation in this communication may contribute to the development or exacerbation of depressive symptoms.

Understanding the relationship between the vagus nerve and depression highlights the potential for interventions targeting the vagal system to alleviate depressive symptoms. Vagus nerve stimulation (VNS) is a treatment approach that involves the use of an implanted device to deliver electrical impulses to the vagus nerve, helping to modulate its activity. VNS has shown promising results in the treatment of treatment-resistant depression and is being investigated for its effectiveness in managing depression.

Other approaches to improving vagal tone and potentially benefiting individuals with depression include relaxation techniques such as deep breathing exercises, meditation, yoga, physical activity, and interventions targeting inflammation reduction, like dietary changes or anti-inflammatory medications.

NOTE: *It's important to note that depression is a complex condition, and the vagus nerve is just one aspect among many involved in its development and maintenance. Treatment for depression often requires a comprehensive approach that involves therapy, medication, lifestyle changes, and support from healthcare professionals.*

6.3 PTSD and the Vagus Nerve

Post-traumatic stress disorder (PTSD) is a psychological wellness condition that can be fostered after somebody has encountered or seen a horrendous mishap. The symptoms of PTSD can include intrusive thoughts or memories of the traumatic event, nightmares, flashbacks, hyperarousal, avoidance of triggers, and heightened anxiety or fear.

Several studies have suggested that there is an intricate relationship between PTSD and the vagus nerve.

Here are some key aspects:

- **Autonomic Nervous System Dysregulation:** PTSD is associated with dysregulation of the autonomic nervous system (ANS), which controls involuntary body functions. The vagus nerve plays a crucial role in the parasympathetic division of the ANS, responsible for the body's rest and digestion response. In individuals with PTSD, there is often a dominance of the sympathetic nervous system (responsible for the fight-or-flight response) over the parasympathetic nervous system. This imbalance can lead to heightened arousal, increased heart rate, and other physiological responses related to anxiety and stress.

- **Heart Rate Variability (HRV):** The vagus nerve is responsible for modulating heart rate variability (HRV), which refers to the variation in the time interval between heartbeats. HRV is an indicator of the body's ability to adapt to stress and regulate the autonomic nervous system. Reduced HRV has been observed in individuals with PTSD, indicating a dysfunction in the vagus nerve's control over heart rate. This reduced HRV may contribute to the persistent state of hyperarousal and anxiety experienced by individuals with PTSD.

- **Inflammation and Immune Response:** The vagus nerve also plays a role in controlling inflammation and immune responses in the body. In individuals with PTSD, there is evidence of increased inflammation markers and alterations in immune function. Dysfunctional vagal activity may contribute to this inflammation and immune dysregulation, leading to various physical health problems often associated with PTSD, such as cardiovascular disease, autoimmune disorders, and gastrointestinal issues.

- **Reversal of the Stress Response:** The vagus nerve activation is closely linked to the activation of the relaxation response, often referred to as the "rest and digest" state. This response is the opposite of the fight-or-flight stress response and is characterized by a decrease in heart rate, blood pressure, and stress hormone levels. In individuals with PTSD, the vagus nerve's ability to activate the relaxation response may be impaired, leading to difficulties in calming down and returning to a state of rest after a traumatic event or trigger.

- **Polyvagal Theory:** The relationship between PTSD and the vagus nerve is further explained by the Polyvagal Theory, proposed by Dr. Stephen Porges. According to this theory, the vagus nerve has two main branches: the ventral vagus and the dorsal vagus. The ventral vagus is associated with social engagement, emotional regulation, and the ability to form safe and secure attachments. The dorsal vagus, on the other hand, is related to a shutdown response, dissociation, and numbing.

In individuals with PTSD, the ventral vagus may be impaired, leading to difficulties in regulating emotions, forming and maintaining relationships, and feeling safe and connected to others. This impairment may contribute to the development and maintenance of PTSD symptoms.

Understanding the relationship between PTSD and the vagus nerve is crucial for the development of effective treatment strategies. Therapies such as biofeedback, heart rate variability training, and vagus nerve stimulation have been explored as potential interventions for PTSD, aiming to modulate vagal activity and restore autonomic balance. These approaches aim to activate the relaxation response, reduce hyperarousal, and alleviate symptoms associated with PTSD.

Overall, the relationship between PTSD and the vagus nerve highlights the complex interplay between the mind and body in the development and maintenance of this mental health condition. Further research is needed to fully understand the mechanisms underlying this relationship and to develop targeted interventions for individuals with PTSD.

6.4 Vagus Nerve Stimulation Therapies for Mental Health

Vagus Nerve Stimulation (VNS) therapies are a form of neuromodulation that involves the electrical stimulation of the vagus nerve. These therapies have shown promise in the treatment of various mental health conditions, including depression, anxiety disorders, post-traumatic stress disorder (PTSD), and epilepsy.

Here is a detailed explanation of Vagus Nerve Stimulation therapies for mental health:

- **Vagus Nerve Stimulation (VNS) Device:** VNS therapy utilizes a small implantable device that is surgically placed under the skin in the chest area. This device is connected to the vagus nerve in the neck through a lead wire, which delivers electrical pulses to the nerve. The device can be programmed and adjusted based on the individual's specific needs.

- **Mechanism of Action:** VNS therapy works by stimulating the vagus nerve, which is a major component of the parasympathetic nervous system. Activation of the vagus nerve releases neurotransmitters such as norepinephrine, serotonin, and gamma-aminobutyric acid (GABA), which are involved in mood regulation, anxiety reduction, and stress response modulation. By modulating these neurotransmitters, VNS therapy aims to normalize brain activity and improve mental health symptoms.

- **Depression Treatment:** VNS therapy has been approved by the U.S. Food and Drug Administration (FDA) for the treatment of treatment-resistant depression. It is used in individuals who have not sufficiently responded to multiple antidepressant medications. The electrical stimulation delivered by the VNS device is thought to increase the availability of neurotransmitters like serotonin and norepinephrine, which are often depleted in individuals with depression. This can help improve mood, reduce depressive symptoms, and enhance overall well-being.

- **Anxiety and PTSD Treatment:** VNS therapy has also shown promise in the treatment of anxiety disorders and PTSD. By stimulating the vagus nerve, this therapy can activate the body's relaxation response and reduce the hyperarousal and anxiety associated with these conditions. It is believed to modulate the autonomic nervous system, regulate heart rate variability, and enhance emotional regulation. While research in this area is still ongoing, early studies have shown positive outcomes in reducing anxiety symptoms and improving quality of life.

- **Epilepsy Treatment:** VNS therapy has been used as an adjunctive treatment for epilepsy, particularly in individuals with drug-resistant seizures. The electrical stimulation provided by the VNS device can help reduce the frequency and severity of seizures. The exact mechanism of action is not fully understood, but it is believed to involve the modulation of abnormal electrical activity in the brain.

- **Side Effects and Safety:** VNS therapy is generally considered safe, but there are some potential side effects associated with the procedure and the device. These can include hoarseness or voice changes, coughing, shortness of breath, difficulty swallowing, neck pain, headache, and nausea. However, most side effects are reported to be mild and temporary. Regular monitoring and follow-up with a healthcare professional are necessary to ensure the safe and effective use of VNS therapy.

- **Ongoing Research and Future Directions:** VNS therapy for mental health conditions is still an area of active research. Researchers are investigating its effectiveness in various populations, exploring optimal stimulation parameters, and identifying potential biomarkers of treatment response. Other forms of non-invasive vagus nerve stimulation, such as transcutaneous vagus nerve stimulation (tVNS), are also being explored as alternative options that do not require surgical implantation.

In conclusion, Vagus Nerve Stimulation therapies offer a promising approach for treating mental health conditions such as depression, anxiety disorders, PTSD, and epilepsy. By modulating the vagus nerve, these therapies aim to restore balance to the autonomic nervous system, enhance mood regulation, and reduce symptoms associated with these conditions. While more research is needed to fully understand the mechanisms of action and optimize treatment protocols, VNS therapy provides a potential avenue for individuals who have not responded to conventional treatments. It is important to consult with a healthcare professional to determine if VNS therapy is appropriate and to discuss the potential benefits and risks specific to each individual's situation.

Chapter Seven

7. Conclusion and Future Directions

In conclusion, the vagus nerve plays a crucial role in regulating various bodily functions and is intricately connected to mental health and well-being. Research on the vagus nerve has highlighted its involvement in the stress response, inflammation, immune function, and emotional regulation.

Vagus nerve stimulation therapies have emerged as a promising approach to treating mental health conditions such as depression, anxiety disorders, PTSD, and epilepsy. These therapies aim to modulate vagal activity and restore autonomic balance, leading to improvements in symptoms and quality of life. While VNS therapy has shown positive outcomes in some individuals, further research is needed to understand the underlying mechanisms, optimal stimulation parameters, and long-term effects.

Future directions in vagus nerve research include exploring non-invasive forms of stimulation, developing personalized treatment approaches, and identifying biomarkers to predict treatment response. Advancements in neuroimaging techniques, such as functional magnetic resonance imaging (fMRI) and electroencephalography (EEG), can provide valuable insights into the effects of vagal stimulation on the brain and help refine treatment protocols.

Moreover, understanding the bidirectional relationship between the vagus nerve and mental health opens up new avenues for integrated treatments. Combining vagus nerve stimulation therapies with psychotherapy, medication, and lifestyle interventions may offer more comprehensive and effective approaches to managing mental health conditions.

Overall, the vagus nerve holds great potential as a target for therapeutic interventions in mental health. Continued research and advancements in this field may lead to more personalized and targeted treatments, improved outcomes, and enhanced understanding of the complex interactions between the mind and body. By harnessing the power of the vagus nerve, we can potentially make significant strides in improving the lives of individuals affected by mental health disorders.

7.1 Summary of Accessing the Healing Power of the Vagus Nerve

Accessing the Healing Power of the Vagus Nerve is a book written by Dr. Walter M. Price that explores the role of the vagus nerve in our overall well-being and healing process. The vagus nerve, also known as the "wandering nerve," extends from the brainstem to various organs in the body, including the heart, lungs, and digestive system. Dr. Walter M. Price explains how stimulating and activating the vagus nerve can have profound effects on our physical and mental health. The book offers practical techniques and exercises to help readers increase vagal tone and promote relaxation, resilience, and healing. It also delves into the connection between the vagus nerve and various health conditions such as anxiety, depression, migraines, and chronic pain. By understanding and accessing the healing power of the vagus nerve,
we can potentially improve our overall well-being and quality of life.

7.2 Potential Areas for Further Research

While the understanding of the vagus nerve's role in health and healing has significantly advanced in recent years, there are still several potential areas for further research. These areas include:

- **Clinical Applications:** Further research is needed to explore the clinical applications of vagus nerve stimulation (VNS) in treating various health conditions. While VNS has been approved for certain conditions like epilepsy and depression, there is potential for its use in other areas such as anxiety disorders, chronic pain, autoimmune diseases, and gastrointestinal disorders.

- **Mechanisms of Action:** Understanding the underlying mechanisms through which vagus nerve stimulation affects various physiological and psychological processes is essential for developing targeted interventions. More research is needed to elucidate the molecular and cellular pathways involved in the vagus nerve's influence on inflammation, immune response, mood regulation, and stress response.

- **Vagal Tone Assessment:** Developing more accurate and accessible methods to assess vagal tone is crucial for monitoring and evaluating interventions targeting the vagus nerve. Traditional methods, such as heart rate variability analysis, could be improved, and new biomarkers might be identified to provide more comprehensive insights into vagal function.

- **Neural Plasticity:** Investigating the vagus nerve's role in neural plasticity, or the brain's ability to reorganize and adapt, is another area of interest. Exploring how VNS can enhance neuroplasticity and promote brain health may have implications for conditions such as stroke recovery, neurodegenerative diseases, and cognitive impairments.

- **Gut-Brain Axis:** Given the extensive network of the vagus nerve connecting the brain with the gut, further research is needed to understand its role in the gut-brain axis. Investigating how vagal signaling influences gut functions, such as digestion, gut microbiota, and intestinal barrier integrity, could provide insights into gastrointestinal disorders, irritable bowel syndrome, and the influence of gut health on mental well-being.

- **Non-Invasive Stimulation Techniques:** While vagus nerve stimulation is currently performed using invasive techniques, exploring non-invasive methods, such as transcutaneous vagus nerve stimulation (tVNS), could open up new possibilities for therapeutic interventions. Further research is needed to compare the efficacy and safety of invasive and non-invasive stimulation techniques and understand their optimal parameters for different health conditions.

- **Individual Variability:** Investigating the individual variability in vagal tone and response to vagus nerve stimulation is crucial for personalizing interventions. Factors such as genetics, lifestyle, and environmental influences may contribute to variations. Further research could help identify biomarkers or predictors of individual vagal responsiveness and tailor interventions accordingly.

- **Long-term Effects:** Studying the long-term effects of vagus nerve stimulation and its impact on overall health and quality of life is essential. Research on the sustainability of the effects, potential side effects, and optimal duration and frequency of stimulation is needed to inform clinical practice and ensure the safety and efficacy of vagus nerve interventions.

Overall, while there has been significant progress in understanding the vagus nerve's role in health and healing, further research in these areas can enhance our understanding of its potential therapeutic applications and pave the path for more targeted interventions.

7.3. Final Thoughts and Recommendations for Vagus Nerve Health

In conclusion, fostering vagus nerve health can have profound benefits for our overall well-being and healing. Here are some final thoughts and recommendations for promoting vagus nerve health:

- **Mindfulness and Relaxation Practices:** Engaging in practices that promote relaxation and reduce stress, such as meditation, deep breathing exercises, and progressive muscle relaxation, can activate the vagus nerve and increase vagal tone.

- **Physical Exercise:** Regular physical exercise has been shown to increase vagal tone, promote cardiovascular health, and improve mood. Incorporating activities like aerobic exercise, yoga, or tai chi into your routine can have positive effects on vagus nerve health.

- **Social Connections:** Cultivating meaningful social connections and engaging in supportive relationships can stimulate the vagus nerve's social engagement system. This includes activities like spending quality time with loved ones, participating in group activities, or joining social clubs.

- **Cold Exposure: Cold** showers or immersions in cold water have been shown to activate the vagus nerve. Gradually exposing yourself to cold temperatures can stimulate the vagus nerve and improve vagal tone.

- **Healthy Diet:** Consuming a diet rich in whole foods, particularly those high in omega-3 fatty acids, probiotics, and antioxidants, can support vagus nerve health. Additionally, avoiding excessive consumption of processed foods, sugar, and inflammatory foods can help maintain a healthy gut and overall vagal function.

- **Sleep Hygiene:** Prioritizing quality sleep and practicing good sleep hygiene can positively impact vagus nerve function. Aim for consistent bedtime routines, a comfortable sleep environment, and sufficient hours of sleep.

- **Vagus Nerve Stimulation Techniques:** Exploring vagus nerve stimulation techniques, such as deep breathing exercises, gargling, humming, or singing, can directly stimulate the vagus nerve and increase vagal tone. Regularly incorporating these practices into your daily routine can have lasting benefits.

- **Seek Professional Guidance:** If you are exploring vagus nerve stimulation therapies, such as VNS devices or neuromodulation techniques, it is crucial to seek guidance from healthcare professionals experienced in this field. They can provide personalized recommendations and ensure these interventions are safe and effective for your specific needs.

NOTE: *Remember that promoting vagus nerve health is a holistic approach, combining various lifestyle factors to optimize overall well-being. However, it is essential to consult with healthcare professionals and listen to your body to determine what strategies work best for you. By nurturing and accessing the healing power of the vagus nerve, we can enhance our ability to heal, recover, and thrive with improved physical and mental health.*

FREQUENTLY ASKED QUESTIONS (FAQs)

Due to its diverse functions, there are several frequently asked questions (FAQs) related to the vagus nerve, which are discussed in detail below:

1. What is the vagus nerve?

The vagus nerve, also known as cranial nerve X or the tenth cranial nerve, is a paired nerve that starts in the brainstem and extends down to the abdomen. It consists of thousands of nerve fibers and branches out to various organs, including the heart, lungs, digestive tract, and vocal cords.

2. What does the vagus nerve do?

The vagus nerve is responsible for regulating numerous bodily functions. It controls the heart rate and blood pressure, stimulates digestion, promotes the release of gastric acid and digestive enzymes, regulates bowel movements, controls the muscles that aid in swallowing and speaking, influences the production of tears and saliva, and has an impact on mood, memory, and overall brain function.

3. How does the vagus nerve affect mental health?

Studies have shown that the vagus nerve plays a crucial role in mental health. It is involved in the regulation of stress response through its connection with the parasympathetic nervous system. Activation of the vagus nerve helps to reduce the release of stress hormones and promotes a state of calm and relaxation. Imbalances or dysfunction of the vagus nerve have been associated with mental health conditions such as anxiety, depression, and PTSD.

4. Can the vagus nerve be stimulated?

Yes, the vagus nerve can be stimulated through various techniques, including vagus nerve stimulation (VNS). VNS involves the use of a device that sends electrical impulses to the vagus nerve, helping to regulate its activity. VNS has been approved by the FDA as a treatment for certain conditions, including epilepsy and treatment-resistant depression. In addition to VNS, certain lifestyle factors such as deep breathing exercises, meditation, yoga, and acupuncture have also been shown to stimulate the vagus nerve.

5. What are the potential benefits of vagus nerve stimulation?

Vagus nerve stimulation has been found to have several potential benefits. It has been shown to reduce the frequency and intensity of seizures in individuals with epilepsy. In the field of mental health, VNS has been found to alleviate symptoms of depression, particularly in individuals who have not responded adequately to other treatments. It has also shown promising results in the treatment of anxiety disorders, PTSD, and chronic pain. Additionally, VNS has been studied in conditions such as obesity, Alzheimer's disease, and even stroke recovery, although more research is needed in these areas.

6. Are there any risks or side effects associated with vagus nerve stimulation?

Like any medical procedure, vagus nerve stimulation does come with potential risks and side effects. The most common side effects include hoarseness, coughing, difficulty swallowing, and shortness of breath. These secondary effects are normally gentle and work over the long haul. Less common but more serious risks include infection at the incision site, nerve damage, or interference with other medical devices such as pacemakers. It is important to discuss the risks and potential benefits with a healthcare professional before considering vagus nerve stimulation.

7. Can I stimulate the vagus nerve naturally?

Yes, there are several natural ways to stimulate the vagus nerve. Deep breathing exercises, such as diaphragmatic breathing or belly breathing, have been shown to activate the vagus nerve and promote relaxation. Meditation, yoga, and tai chi are practices that can help stimulate the vagus nerve through their focus on slow, deep breathing and relaxation techniques. Cold exposure, such as taking cold showers or immersing your face in cold water, can also activate the vagus nerve. Chewing gum, singing, and laughing are other activities that can stimulate the vagus nerve.

8. Can vagus nerve stimulation help with weight loss?

There is some evidence suggesting that vagus nerve stimulation may have a positive impact on weight loss. The theory is that VNS can help regulate appetite and reduce food cravings, leading to better control over food intake. However, more research is needed to fully understand the effects of VNS on weight loss and its long-term sustainability.

9. Can damage or dysfunction of the vagus nerve be treated?

In some cases, damage or dysfunction of the vagus nerve may be treatable. This depends on the underlying cause and extent of the damage. Vagus nerve injuries caused by trauma or surgical procedures may sometimes require surgical repair. Vagus nerve stimulation is also a potential treatment option for certain conditions associated with vagus nerve dysfunction, such as epilepsy or treatment-resistant depression. In cases where the vagus nerve cannot be fully repaired or stimulated, other treatment modalities may be used to manage symptoms and improve overall well-being.

10. Can I increase my vagal tone?

Yes, it is possible to increase vagal tone, which refers to the activity and responsiveness of the vagus nerve. Increasing vagal tone is associated with improved overall health and well-being. Some ways to increase vagal tone include regular exercise, especially aerobic activities, as well as practices that promote relaxation and stress reduction, such as deep breathing exercises, meditation, and yoga. Adequate sleep, a healthy diet, and maintaining social connections have also been found to positively influence vagal tone.